Dysmenorrhea and Menorrhagia

Roger P. Smith

Dysmenorrhea and Menorrhagia

A Clinician's Guide

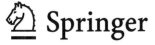 Springer

Roger P. Smith
Florida Atlantic University
Boca Raton, Florida, USA

Additional material to this book can be downloaded from http://extras.springer.com

ISBN 978-3-319-89126-2   ISBN 978-3-319-71964-1   (eBook)
https://doi.org/10.1007/978-3-319-71964-1

Printed on acid-free paper

This Springer imprint is published by Springer Nature
The registered company is Springer International Publishing AG
The registered company address is: Gewerbestrasse 11, 6330 Cham, Switzerland

Contents

Chapter 1
The Physiology of Menstruation

1.1 Topic Overview

Only humans, closely related primates, some species of bats, and elephant shrews (Fig. 1.1) visibly menstruate. The processes that drive the monthly maturation, slough, and renewal of the endometrium that results in menses are ultimately orchestrated by a complex interaction of hormones, tissues, and molecular signaling, all designed to ensure the possibility of securing a pregnancy should a timely mating occur. Menstrual pain and excessive menstrual bleeding are both extremes of a normal continuum. Understanding their development requires a familiarity with the processes that create the normal menstrual cycle. This discussion will focus primarily on the uterus, leaving many of nuances of the complex interactions of the hypothalamus, pituitary, and ovary to others.

Fig. 1.1 A male black and rufous elephant shrew (*Rhynchocyon petersi*) at the National Zoo in Washington, DC

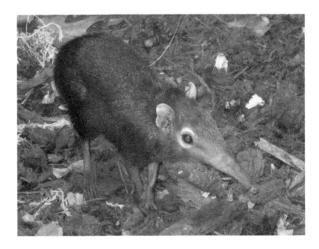

© Springer International Publishing AG 2018
R.P. Smith, *Dysmenorrhea and Menorrhagia*,
https://doi.org/10.1007/978-3-319-71964-1_1

1.2   Major Players

Without the active presence and participation of the hypothalamus, pituitary, and ovary (with its compliment of oocytes and associated cells), the passive uterus would have no cyclic function, no menses, and no menstrual dysfunction. While the anatomy and complex functioning of these tissues are beyond the scope of this text, the cyclic interaction between hypothalamic gonadotropin-releasing hormone (GnRH), the pituitary gonadotropins follicle-stimulating hormone (FSH) and luteinizing hormone (LH), and the ovarian sex steroid hormones estradiol and progesterone drives the endometrial changes responsible for both normal and dysfunctional menstruation. Through positive and negative feedback loops, these hormones stimulate ovulation, facilitate implantation of the fertilized ovum, or bring about menstruation.

The elements required for a successful menstrual cycle can be broadly classified into tissues and hormones: Tissues that support, contain, and respond to the signals that facilitate the maturation and release of the gamete (oocyte), will harbor a conceptus, and provide the needed sequencing controls; and hormones that coordinate functions between cells, structures, and organs to ensure the effective timing of the needed changes.

1.2.1   The Tissues

The organ directly associated with menstrual pain and heavy menstrual bleeding is, of course, the uterus. It is the location of the monthly changes in preparation for a possible pregnancy, and the renewal that occurs in the absence of a conception. Indeed, the endometrium is the only tissue in the body in which the regular, periodic occurrence of necrosis and desquamation is a sign of health rather than of disease. The normal ebb and flow of estrogen and progesterone, through a monthly cycle, first builds up and then takes away, in regular sequence, the support of the endometrium. Menstrual flow that is characterized by repeated regularity in timing, amount, and duration of bleeding, documents a normal and ordered chain of endocrine events for that individual.

The uterus begins to develop at about 4–6 weeks after conception, when the two sets of paired genital ducts, the mesonephric (Wolffian) ducts and the paramesonephric (Müllerian) ducts, develop. Derived from the evaginations of the coelomic epithelium, the paramesonephric ducts form on each side of the mesonephric ducts. For each duct, the invagination fuses to form a tube: The more cephalad ends open directly into the future peritoneal cavity, while the distal ends grow caudally, fusing in the lower midline at approximately the eighth week of development to form the uterovaginal primordium. These nascent structures are destined to form the uterine tubes, the uterus, and the proximal four fifths of the vagina. When the two paramesonephric ducts fuse, two peritoneal folds are brought together. This creates the

Fig. 1.2 The ration of cervical length to uterine body length is roughly 1:1 before puberty. After puberty, this ratio becomes 2:1 or greater

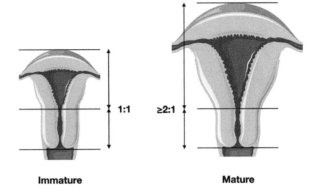

Immature   **Mature**

broad ligaments of the uterus. Ultimately, the mesonephric tubules degenerate into a series of tiny vestigial, epithelial-lined cysts (Gartner's duct cysts), which may be found from the broad ligament to the vaginal vestibule.

Through the seventh month of fetal life, the uterus grows in proportion to the rest of the body. Thereafter, an acceleration in growth takes place in response to the high levels of estrogens transferred across the placenta from the maternal circulation. Following birth, the infant's uterus shrinks slightly due to the abrupt withdrawal of these maternal hormones. This withdrawal can, uncommonly, be sufficient to result in vaginal spotting or frank bleeding. Before puberty, the length of the cervix and the uterine body are approximately equal; after puberty, the ratio of the body to the cervix is between 2:1 and 3:1. In the nulliparous adult, the uterus is approximately 7–8 cm long and 4–5 cm wide at the widest part (Fig. 1.2).

The wall of the uterus is made up of a complexly interdigitated network of smooth muscle fibers and vascular structures, covered by peritoneum, that houses and supports the endometrium and endometrial cavity. The cavity of the uterine body is not a true cavity, but rather a flattened triangular potential space. The fallopian tubes open into its basal angles, with the cervix at the apex. The external longitudinal and internal circular smooth muscle fibers in the tubes are confluent with those in the uterus, spiraling around the uterus in both clockwise and counterclockwise directions (Fig. 1.3).

While a true pacemaker for uterine contractions is lacking, evidence supports both a tubal source and a wandering pacemaker system of independent foci of initiator signals with strong interconnections between the cells through cellular gap junctions. The most dramatic manifestation of these rhythmic contractions is the process of labor, but some level of contractile activity is always present. The amplitude and frequency of smooth muscle contractions are related to ovarian activity, with contractions occurring with greater force and frequency during the preovulatory peak of estrogen production and, under the influence of prostaglandins produced from the sloughed endometrium, during menstruation. The contractions found during menstruation aid in clearing menstrual blood and endometrial remnants from the uterine cavity.

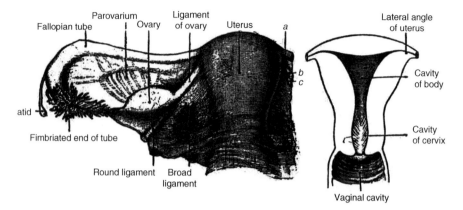

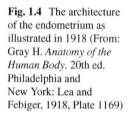

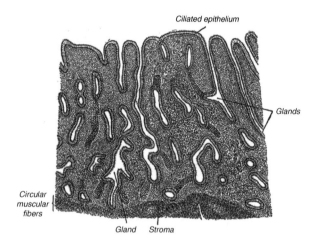

Fig. 1.3 The general anatomy of the uterus (From: A. F. Dixon, Cunningham's *Text-book of Anatomy – Encyclopædia Britannica* (11th ed.), v. 23, 1911, "Reproductive System, in Anatomy," p. 132, Fig. 6)

Fig. 1.4 The architecture of the endometrium as illustrated in 1918 (From: Gray H. *Anatomy of the Human Body*. 20th ed. Philadelphia and New York: Lea and Febiger, 1918, Plate 1169)

The lining of the uterus (endometrium) is made up of two layers defined less by structure than by function: the basal layer (the deepest third of the endometrium) and a functional layer. It is the functional layer, adjacent to the uterine cavity, that thickens in response to estrogen and then is sloughed during menstruation. The basal layer, adjacent to the myometrium and below the functional layer, is not shed during the menstrual cycle and is the source of the regrown functional layer following menstruation (Fig. 1.4).

The endometrium consists of a single layer of columnar epithelium plus the stroma that provides support. The connective tissue stroma also varies in thickness in response to estrogen and progesterone. Simple tubular glands reach from the endometrial surface to the base of the stroma, which also carries a rich supply of spiral arteries. The regrowth of the endometrium following menstruation is under the control of estrogen, while the conversion to a secretory endometrium is under the influence of progesterone. This conversion can only occur if there has been

adequate estrogen priming and growth. In the absence of elevated levels of progesterone, the endometrium remains thinner and may eventually become sessile. When
this occurs, both dysmenorrhea and menorrhagia are less likely.

The secretory endometrium is characterized by an endometrial stroma that
becomes loose and edematous. Blood vessels entering the endometrium become
thickened and twisted, and the endometrial glands, which were straight and tubular,
become tortuous. Increased production of glycogen by the glandular cells is apparent, as glycogen vacuoles accumulate within the glandular cells, migrate to the
luminal surface, and disgorge their content into the gland lumen.

The arcuate uterine arteries, which arise from the ascending and descending
branches of the uterine arteries, circle the uterus just beneath the peritoneal surface.
Radial branches arise at intervals and penetrate directly inward through the myometrium to the endometrium. Before entering the endometrium, the terminal branches
of the radials divide into two distinct types of arteriole: straight and spiral arterioles
(Figs. 1.5 and 1.6).

The short, straight arterioles supply only the deeper third of the endometrium,
ending in a horizontal arborization. These arterioles are not affected by cyclic hor-

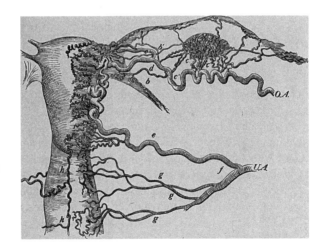

Fig. 1.5 An 1898 view of
the vascular supply of the
uterus: OA, ovarian artery;
b, artery of the round
ligament; b, branch to the
tube; c, c, c, branches to
the ovary; d, continuation
of main trunk; e, branch to
the cornu; U.A., uterine
artery; e, main trunk; f,
bifurcation; g, vaginal
branches; k, vaginal branch
from the cervical artery.
(From: Hirst BC. *A
Textbook of Obstetrics*.
Philadelphia: Saunders,
1898, p. 33, Fig. 19)

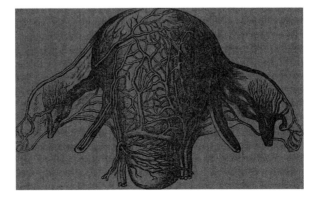

Fig. 1.6 The rich vascular
network of anastomotic
vessels supplying the body
of the uterus is seen in this
1844 illustration. (From:
Dunglinson, R. *Human
physiology with Upwards
of Three Hundred
Illustrations (Volume 2)*.
Philadelphia: Lea and
Blanchard, 1844, p. 417,
Fig. 238)

monal changes, maintaining a continuous circulation to the basal epithelial layers. As a result, the basal layer is continuously nourished and left intact during menstruation, to provide the glandular remnants from which will regrowth the entire epithelial thickness during the intermenstrual period.

In contrast, the spiral arterioles reach to the surface of the endometrium and undergo marked changes in response to hormonal variations through the normal menstrual cycle. Branches are given off that invest glands and supply the stroma. In the superficial layer, a diffuse arteriovenous capillary network terminates in venous lakes or sinusoids. This complicated vascular pattern, unique to the endometrium, was once believed to be the mainspring of the processes that enact the rhythmic necrosis and bleeding that is menstruation. Despite this rich blood supply, the average blood loss during menstruation is 35 mL, with 10–80 mL considered normal.

To supply the hormonal ebb and flow necessary for these uterine changes, the hypothalamus, pituitary, and ovaries must be intact and functioning. The hypothalamus serves as the pulse generator of the reproductive clock, the anterior pituitary the source of the gonadotropins FSH and LH, and the ovary the focus of the ovulation process and the prime producer of estrogens and progestogens.

1.2.2   The Hormones

The interactions of the hypothalamus, pituitary, and ovary (the "hypothalamic-pituitary-ovarian axis") orchestrate the menstrual cycle. Two anterior pituitary gonadotropins and two ovarian steroids are primarily involved in the periodic occurrence of menstruation: The pituitary contributes follicle-stimulating hormone and luteinizing hormone, while the ovary secretes beta-estradiol and progesterone. Other signaling molecules, such as gonadotropin-releasing hormone, inhibin B, and activin, have active roles to play in the process of ovulatory cycling, but an extended discussion of their functions is beyond the scope of this discussion (Fig. 1.7).

The median preoptic area of the hypothalamus is sensitive to the circulating levels of estrogen, inhibin A, inhibin B, and to a lesser extent, progesterone. In response to this feedback, GnRH (a decapeptide) is secreted in a pulsatile manner from the arcuate nucleus of the hypothalamus. The secreted GnRH reaches the anterior pituitary gland through the hypothalamic-pituitary portal plexus where it controls the production and release of FSH and LH. The release of FSH and LH requires the pulsatile secretion of GnRH at 70- to 90-min intervals. Disruptions in this pulsatile timing will result in ovulatory dysfunction, anovulation, and amenorrhea. It is the emergence of this rhythmic process that underlies and drives the transitions of puberty. Low-frequency GnRH pulses are required for FSH release, whereas high-frequency GnRH pulses stimulate LH release in a one-to-one manner. Unlike in men who have a constant frequency of GnRH pulses, in women, the frequency of the GnRH pulses varies during the menstrual cycle, and there is a large surge of GnRH just before ovulation.

Fig. 1.7 The
hypothalamus, pituitary,
and ovaries communicate
with each other through a
combination of positive
(FSH and LH) and
negative (estrogen and, to a
lesser extent, progesterone)
feedback interactions (see
text)

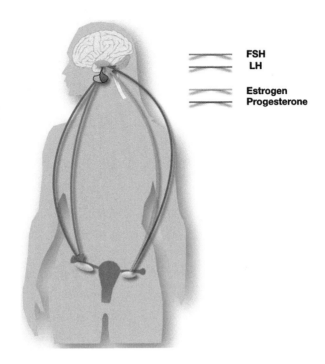

FSH
LH

Estrogen
Progesterone

Both FSH and LH are glycoprotein heterodimers, made up of two polypeptide
units, alpha and beta, that are non-covalently associated. Their structures are similar
to those of thyroid-stimulating hormone (TSH) and human chorionic gonadotropin
(hCG). The alpha subunits of these glycoproteins are identical and consist of about
92 amino acids in humans; it is the beta subunits that vary, with 118 amino acids for
FSH and 120 amino acids for LH. The molecular weight of FSH is 35.5 kDa, while
that of LH is roughly 30 kDa. In the body, the biologic half-life of LH is 20 min,
whereas that of FSH is 3–4 h. Both hormones are produced by gonadotropic cells in
the anterior pituitary gland under the control of the gonadotropin-releasing hormone
made in the hypothalamus (Fig. 1.8).

The magnitude of secretion and the rates of secretion of FSH and/or LH are
determined largely by the levels of ovarian steroid hormones and other ovarian factors such as inhibins A and B, activin, and follistatin. When there is a relative estrogen deficiency, as in the last few days prior to menstruation and the early follicular
phase, the principal gonadotropin secreted is FSH. Because the ovary responds to
FSH secretion with estradiol production, there is increasing negative feedback on
the pituitary. This rising estradiol inhibits FSH secretion and facilitates LH secretion by modulating the pulsatile secretion of GnRH (Fig. 1.9).

For simplicity, the bulk of the estrogen and progesterone production involved
with cyclic menstruation can be treated as ovarian in origin. In humans, there are
three main types of estrogens: estrone (E_1), estradiol (E_2), and estriol (E_3). At equal
concentrations, E_2 has a stronger biological effect than E_1, which is more powerful

Fig. 1.8 A three-dimensional rendering of the molecular structure of the beta polypeptide of follicle-stimulating hormone (FSH)

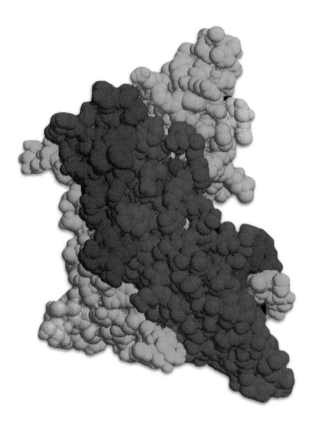

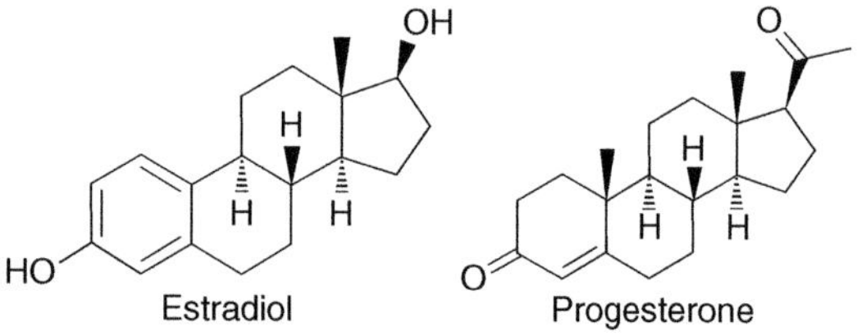

Fig. 1.9 The molecular structures of estradiol and progesterone

Estradiol   Progesterone

than E_3. Influenced by FSH levels, estradiol is produced by the enzymatic conversion of androgens (androstenedione and testosterone), through aromatase activity. The conversion of these androgens to E_2 occurs in the granulosa cells of the follicle using substrates made by the adjacent theca cells. The substrate androgens are produced locally by the theca cells, under the influence of LH, using cholesterol as their substrate. This complex interaction of the theca and granulosa cells under the separate influences of FSH and LH (respectively) has been referred to as the "two-cell model" of estrogen production. In other tissues, such as fat or the adrenal gland, a two-cell process is not required for this conversion (Fig. 1.10).

Binding of FSH to granulosa cell surface receptors causes granulosa cell proliferation, increased binding of FSH, and increased production of estradiol, creating a

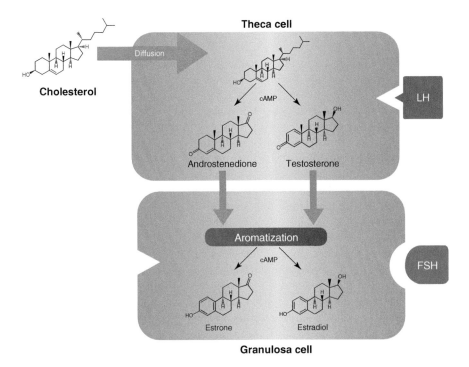

Fig. 1.10 Ovarian estrogen production involves the interactions of the theca and granulosa cells under the separate influence of LH and FSH. Cholesterol that diffuses into the theca cells is metabolized, in the presence of cyclic adenosine monophosphate (cAMP), into the intermediates androstenedione and testosterone. These then undergo aromatization to become estrone and estradiol, respectively

self-reinforcing loop that results in the emergence of a dominant follicle: The follicle with the greatest number of granulosa cells, FSH receptors, and highest estradiol production becomes the dominant follicle from which ovulation will occur. Receptors for LH on the granulosa cell eventually convert the cellular machinery to facilitate the formation of progesterone.

In the middle of the menstrual cycle, it is the LH peak which induces biochemical and phenotypic changes in granulosa cells (luteinization), enabling granulosa cell production of progesterone. Progesterone transforms the endometrium, already stimulated by E_2, into a secretory mucosa, which can support the implantation of a fertilized ovum. Progesterone also inhibits uterine contractions, facilitating sperm and conceptus migration, and the process of implantation. If pregnancy does not occur, the corpus luteum undergoes involution, menstruation begins, and the cycle repeats.

Because of tissue necrosis and the liberation of phospholipids from deteriorating cell walls, there is an acceleration of prostaglandin formation at the time of menstruation. These prostaglandins are responsible for stimulating the rhythmic contraction of the uterus that helps expel the endometrial debris and blood that make up menstrual fluid. The production and function of these critical signaling molecules (autacoids) are the subject of a separate chapter.

1.3   The Sequence of Events

Menarche, the first menstrual cycle, heralds the onset of adult reproductive function, which continues until menopause, when the major part of ovarian function ceases. Absent the hiatus afforded by pregnancies, between menarche and menopause, the hormonal ballet of cyclic menstruation occurs.

At the onset of menstrual flow (defined as day 1), production of estrogen and progesterone is low, but that of FSH is high. High levels of FSH stimulate the rapid conversion of pre-granulosa cells, making up the primordial follicles, into proliferating and hormonally active granulosa cells. The increase in FSH begins approximately 2 days before the onset of menstruation, when the lowest levels of estrogen and progesterone are found, thus releasing the negative feedback on the hypothalamus and from the hypothalamus to the anterior pituitary. Through a maturation process that takes 375 days, several follicles will have developed enough to respond with this transformation in answer to the elevated FSH levels. During this evolution, pre-granulosa cells are prompted by FSH to become granulosa cells, which begin secreting estradiol. In addition, FSH stimulates mitosis of the granulosa cells, thereby increasing the number of granulosa cells surrounding the oocyte (Fig. 1.11).

Estradiol, itself, also contributes to this self-propagating process by stimulating the expression of LH receptors on the theca cell's surface, increasing secretion of androgen precursors, which are then converted to estradiol in granulosa cells. This upregulation of LH cell surface receptors and hormone production prepares the granulosa and theca cells for progesterone synthesis after ovulation. The early rise in estrogen, seen by about day 4 or 5 of the cycle, shuts off menstrual bleeding and triggers endometrial regeneration through the mitogenic effects of the estrogen.

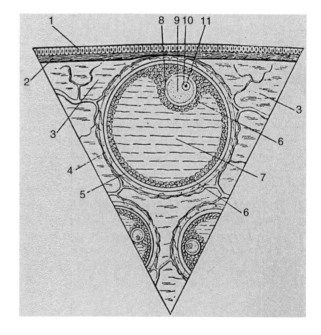

Fig. 1.11 A view of the granulosa cell layer surrounding the follicle from 1889. (1, Epithelial covering of ovary. 2, Tunica albuginea (fibrous). 3, Different parts of stroma. 4, Graafian follicle (tunica fibrosa). 5, Graafian vesicle or ovisac. 6, Tunica granulosa. 7, Liquor folliculi. 8, Vitelline membrane or zona pellucida. 9, Granular vitellus or yolk. 10, Germinal vesicle. 11, Germinal spot). (From: King, AFA. *A Manual of Obstetrics*. Philadelphia: Lea Brothers & Co., 1889, p. 62, Fig. 14)

The progressively increasing effects of estrogen on its own production and follicle development mean that most new follicles have a relatively short life if they miss out on this wave of proliferation and production. Without sufficient receptors and differentiation to participate in this self-reinforcing process, their granulosa cells and ovum degenerate, leaving an atretic follicle. A few continue to enlarge, but in most cycles, only one emerges as the mature Graafian follicle that ruptures (ovulation) about cycle day 14 (Fig. 1.12).

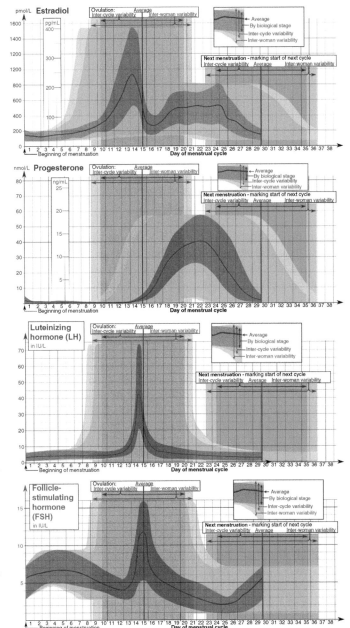

Fig. 1.12 Changes in key hormonal level across time and between women. (From: Häggström, M. Reference ranges for estradiol, progesterone, luteinizing hormone and follicle-stimulating hormone during the menstrual cycle. *WikiJournal of Medicine* 2014:**1**(1).)

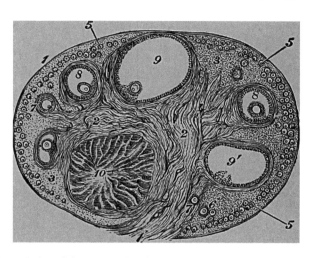

Fig. 1.13 The evolution of the ovarian follicle from primordial to corpus luteum, as shown in 1905. (1, outer covering; 1′, ovarian pedicle; 2, central stroma; 3, peripheral stroma; 4, blood vessels; 5, Graafian follicles in their earliest stage; 6, 7, 8, more advanced follicles; 9, an almost mature follicle; 9′, follicle from which the ovum has escaped; 10, corpus luteum). (From: Findley, P. *The diagnosis of diseases of women.* 2nd ed. Philadelphia and New York: Lea Brothers & Co, 1905, p. 410, Fig. 170)

It is the continued production of estrogen, progesterone, and inhibin by the ovary and follicle that suppresses the hypothalamus, decreasing its GnRH production, which, in turn, decreases the release of FSH and increases the release of LH from the anterior pituitary. (During the early follicular portion of the cycle, the FSH to LH ratio is >1, but as the cycle progresses, the FSH to LH ratio becomes <1, demonstrating this modulating feedback effect of estradiol on the pituitary.) The withdrawal of the FSH stimulus slows follicular development and prevents other emerging follicles from maturing and releasing their eggs. This self-limiting process generally insures that there is only one egg, which can be fertilized each month. Failure of this inhibition, or the near simultaneous rupture of more than one follicle, can result in fraternal twinning or higher-order pregnancies (Fig. 1.13).

The early proliferative endometrium is characterized by a thin surface epithelium, and sparse glands, which are thin and straight. Few mitoses are seen and there is little pseudostratification of gland nuclei. As proliferation continues, the glands become more tortuous and the surface epithelium becomes tall and columnar. This reaches a maximum 1–2 days before ovulation occurs. At this point, the glands may show numerous mitoses with moderate or marked pseudostratification. Dense stroma is found at this stage.

The spiral arterioles of the endometrium undergo extreme lengthening during the proliferative phase of the cycle, outstripping the stromal elements, which proliferate, but at a much slower rate. Because of this difference in growing speed, the spiral arteries are thrown into complex kinks and coils, giving them their name. This coiling would be even more dramatic were it not for the simultaneous accumulation of supportive interstitial fluid that develops during the first preovulatory peak of estrogen production.

Through about day 12 of the cycle, the secretion of FSH decreases with the increase of follicular estrogen production suppressing GnRH production by the hypothalamus. Although follicular growth beyond the stage of antrum formation must be initiated by the pituitary and continues dependent on this stimulus for the first week or so of the cycle, after about cycle day 8, the further development is autonomous as noted above. A surge of LH (and to a lesser extent FSH) also reflects this rising estrogenic tide, and it provides the endocrine trigger for ovulation.

The early presence of FSH, stimulating mitosis of granulosa cells and production of estradiol, also induces additional LH receptors on the surface of the granulosa cells and theca cells. With the LH surge at the time of ovulation, these LH receptors bind LH and convert the enzymatic machinery of the cells to facilitate production of progesterone. After ovulation, estrogen levels drop slightly during a few days of lag between the functional peak of the mature follicle and that of the fully developed corpus luteum. Some uterine spotting or even bleeding for a day or two is not rare ("mid-cycle bleeding") due to this brief reduction of hormonal support.

The production of progesterone begins approximately 24 h before ovulation and rises rapidly thereafter, reaching a maximal production of 3–4 days after ovulation. Robust production is maintained for approximately 11 days following ovulation unless supported by the presence of human chorionic gonadotropin (hCG) from an implanted fertilized ovum. Progesterone has negative feedback on pituitary secretion of both FSH and LH. Therefore, during the luteal phase of the cycle, both FSH and LH are suppressed to low levels, insuring that should a conception occur, follicular development and further ovulations will be suppressed. (This is the primary mechanism of action of both combination hormonal contraceptives and progesterone-only contraceptive methods.) As the corpus luteum fails and progesterone secretion diminishes, FSH begins to emerge from this suppression and rises to prepare for the next reproductive cycle (Fig. 1.14).

The effects of progesterone can be detected by secretory changes in the endometrium within 48 h after ovulation. Progesterone is not a mitogen but causes differentiation of

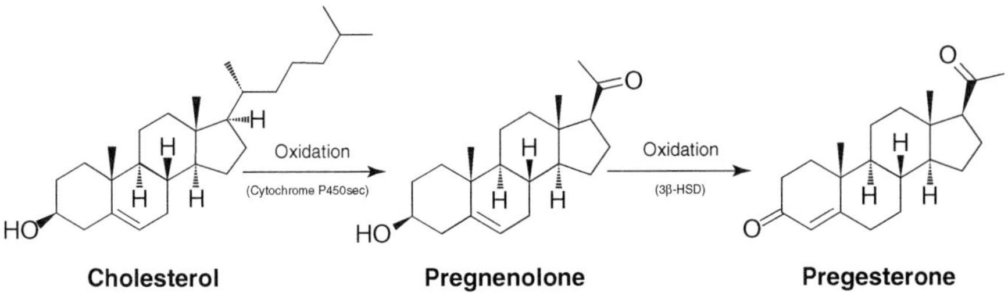

Cholesterol	Pregnenolone	Pregesterone

Fig. 1.14 Cholesterol undergoes double oxidation through cholesterol side-chain cleavage enzymes in the mitochondria to produce pregnenolone. This reaction is catalyzed by cytochrome P450scc. The conversion of pregnenolone to progesterone takes place in two steps involving enzymes bound to the smooth endoplasmic reticulum: the 3β-hydroxyl group is oxidized to a keto group, and second, the double bond is moved to C4, from C5 through a reaction catalyzed by 3β-hydroxysteroid dehydrogenase/δ^{5-4}-isomerase. Pregnenolone and progesterone can be further metabolized to a number of androgens (*3β-HSD* 3-beta-hydroxysteroid dehydrogenase)

Fig. 1.15 A low-power view of premenstrual endometrium. At the bottom is the muscle of the uterine wall, sharply demarcated from the endometrium. The glands in the deepest part of the endometrium are small, and their epithelial cells low. At the middle of the endometrium, the glands are dilated, the epithelium wavy, and the epithelial cells swollen and actively secreting mucus. The stroma cells are larger and lie further apart. On the right, the dilatation of the blood vessels can be seen. Near the top the glands have the same characteristic as at the middle, but there is more edema of the stroma. (From: Graves WD. *Gynecology*. Philadelphia: Saunders, 1918, p. 25, Fig. 1)

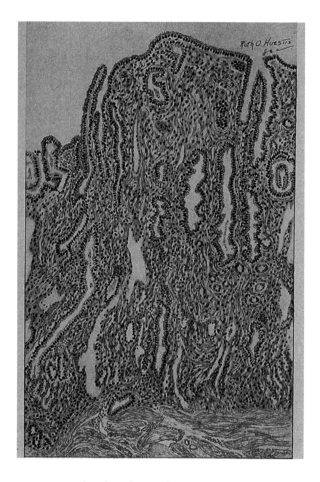

the tissues that have been estrogen primed and contain progesterone receptors. Progesterone from the corpus luteum causes the glands of the endometrium to become secretory, vessels become tortuous, and vascular lakes appear in the edematous stroma. The endometrial glands, which were straight and tubular in the proliferative phase of the endometrium, also become tortuous and contain secretory material within their lumen. Subnuclear vacuoles may be seen. Secretion into the lumen of the glands reaches its peak at about the sixth postovulatory day. These changes prepare the endometrium to support the implantation of a fertilized egg (Fig. 1.15).

A second period of endometrial fluid retention is found at the height of progesterone production. As a result, the spiral arteries are somewhat stretched during the time of greatest luteal activity. Under the influence of estrogen and progesterone, the growth and the secretory activity of the endometrium progress continuously through cycle day 25 or 26. In the absence of a fertilized, implanted ovum, the corpus luteum begins to degenerate just before the end of the menstrual cycle. This is accompanied by the fall in blood levels of estrogen and progesterone and, consequently, by a resorption of the interstitial fluid. The endometrium shrinks, becomes denser, and forces the spiral arteries to kink and "buckle."

From 4 to 24 h preceding the onset of menstrual bleeding, intense vasoconstriction is seen. The vasoconstriction, together with the antecedent buckling, was thought to lead to severe ischemia and necrosis of the superficial parts of the endometrium, progressing to the actual desquamation of menstruation. The actual initiation of menstrual sloughing occurs because of direct enzymatic digestion of the superficial tissues, which is hormonally dependent; progesterone withdrawal induces the expression of matrix metalloproteinases (MMPs) 1, 3, and 9 and releases suppression of prostaglandin synthesis. (Matrix metalloproteinases 1, 3, and 9 degrade the extravascular and stromal matrix.) At the end of this digestive process, vasoconstriction of vessels becomes profound, and reepithelialization of endometrial tissues takes place, generated from the undisturbed basal layers (Fig. 1.16).

Vasoconstriction is critical to the cessation of bleeding from the denuded endometrium because the normal clotting mechanism, involving platelet-fibrin plugs, is absent in the endometrium. This critical vasoconstriction is driven by the presence of thromboxane A_2 (TXA_2) and prostaglandin $F_{2\alpha}$ ($PGF_{2\alpha}$) produced by intense

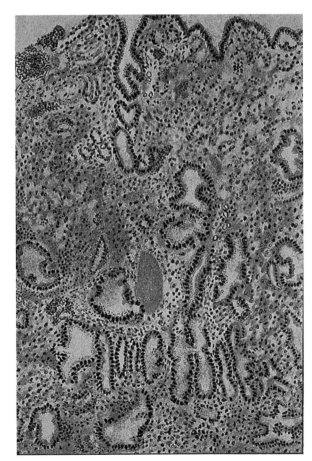

Fig. 1.16 A low-power view of the menstruating endometrium. At the top left, the surface epithelium is gone. The glands throughout have discharged their contents and collapsed. The epithelial cells are still swollen. The stroma is very edematous and infiltrated with blood, especially on the left. At the bottom, the glands are still somewhat dilated, but there is very little edema of the stroma and straight direction. When the bleeding has ceased, the edema of the stroma disappears. (From: Graves WD. *Gynecology*. Philadelphia: Saunders, 1918, p. 29, Fig. 5)

cyclooxygenase activity in the upper endometrium. The balance of the strongly vasoconstrictive TXA_2, the related vasodilators prostacyclin (PGI_2) and prostaglandin E_2 (PGE_2), appears to be critical to regulating total blood loss during menstruation. These prostanoids have very short half-lives, 40 s and 3 min respectively for thromboxane and prostacyclin, limiting their action to the local tissues. Adding to the effects of TXA_2, are the endothelins of the vessels themselves. Endothelin-1, the most powerful vasoconstrictor yet discovered, has been demonstrated in human endometrium. Though vasoconstriction provides the main hemostatic mechanism for the initial 24–48 h after the onset of menstruation, subsequent blood loss is controlled by regeneration of the endometrial vessels and surrounding tissues.

The lifespan of the corpus luteum ends approximately 9–11 days after ovulation. If conception does not take place, the fate of the corpus luteum is involution. It is during this regressive phase that the decrease of estrogen and progesterone production prompts a new output of pituitary gonadotropins, producing stimulation for a new crop of ovarian follicles, and a new ovulatory growth cycle is once more initiated. Thus, during menstruation, follicular growth has already been initiated for the next cycle.

1.4   The Perception of Pain

For a minority of women, even the mild, irregular uterine contractions that occur throughout the menstrual cycle are perceptible. (The mid-cycle pain occasionally associated with ovulation is caused by stretch of the peritoneum investing the ovary, and not through the same mechanisms or pathways as contraction-generated neural impulses, which underlie menstrual pain.) Because of the neural pathways involved, most perceptions originating from the pelvic viscera are poorly mapped. Because visceral structures do not have cortical representations, the sensation of pain is generally referred to superficial areas of the body. These areas are usually those with similar innervation as that of the viscus. Hence, the complaint of pain may be similar for widely different etiologies. This lack of specificity results in most menstrual symptoms being broadly described as being in the lower abdomen or low back.

The pelvic organs are mainly supplied by the autonomic nervous system. The sympathetic portion of the autonomic nervous system originates in the thoracic and lumbar portions of the spinal cord, with sympathetic ganglia located adjacent to the central nervous system. The parasympathetic portion originates in cranial nerves and the middle three sacral segments of the cord. Here the ganglia are located near the visceral organs. Although the fibers of these two systems frequently intermingle in the same peripheral nerves, their physiologic actions are usually antagonistic: Sympathetic fibers produce smooth muscle contraction (including vasoconstriction), whereas parasympathetic fibers cause the opposite effect.

Pain input from the pelvic organs comes primarily by way of small afferent fibers that accompany sympathetic nerves. These enter the spinal cord at T_{10}, T_{11}, T_{12}, and the L_1 levels. Their course carries them through the uterine, cervical, and pelvic

Fig. 1.17 The nerve supply of the uterus as shown in 1846. (From: Beck TS, 'On the Nerves of the Uterus', in *Philosophical Transactions of the Royal Society of London*, 1846, vol. 1 Plate XII, engraving referring to page 233: female urogenital system, Wellcome Library, London)

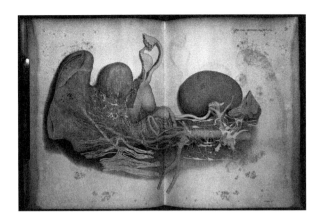

plexuses, the hypogastric nerve, the superior hypogastric plexus (the presacral nerve), as well as the lumbar and lower lumbar sympathetic chain. Exact pathways are difficult to trace with certainty, making any therapeutic approach to blocking pain sensation difficult. Once afferent fibers pass through the dorsal roots and enter the spinal cord, the signal they carry is subject to modulation at the local, segmental, and supraspinal levels. It is thought that it is at this level that interventions such as transcutaneous electrical nerve stimulation (TENS) have its effect (Fig. 1.17).

Key Points
- The cyclic changes in the endometrium that constitute the menstrual cycle are predominately under the control of estrogen and progesterone.
- Estrogen and progesterone are primarily produced in the follicle and corpus luteum under the influence of the pituitary hormones FSH and LH.
- Pituitary production of FSH and LH is controlled by feedback mechanisms through estrogen and progesterone themselves acting on the hypothalamus.
- The secretory changes that the endometrium undergoes to prepare for a possible implantation require estrogen priming.
- In the absence of elevated levels of progesterone, the endometrium remains thinner and may eventually become sessile.

Additional Resources

For excellent images and an overview of the anatomy of the female reproductive organs:
Smith RP, Turek P. The Netter Collection of medical illustrations: reproductive system. Philadelphia, PA: Elsevier—Global Medicine Group; 2011.
For a review of the structure and functions of FSH and LH:
Padmanabhan V, Karsch FJ, Lee JS. Hypothalamic, pituitary and gonadal regulation of FSH. Reprod Suppl. 2002;59:67–82.
Pierce JG, Parsons TF. Glycoprotein hormones: structure and function. Annu Rev Biochem. 1981;**50**(1):465–95. https://doi.org/10.1146/annurev.bi.50.070181.002341.
An excellent overview of the role of prostaglandins in menstruation can be found at:
Drife JO, Calder AA, editors. Prostaglandins and the uterus. London: Springer-Verlag; 1992.

Chapter 2
Scope of the Problems

2.1 Topic Overview

Pain, whether acute, chronic, or recurring, is a major source of morbidity and disability, costing uncounted billions of dollars annually in both direct and indirect costs. The diagnosis and treatment of pain have taken on increased importance in recent years and are now identified as a "vital sign" by the Joint Commission on Accreditation Healthcare Organizations (JCAHO). The treatment of both acute and chronic pain with opiate pain relievers has led to a national crisis over opiate abuse and dependence. For women, pelvic pain is by far the most common type of pain complaint for which treatment is sought [1, 2]. The cyclic pain of dysmenorrhea has been estimated to affect up to 80% of women at some point in their life, with 50% or more experiencing it on a regular basis. Without access to effective treatments, this scope of incapacity should be intolerable to any developed society (Fig. 2.1).

Menstrual periods that involve excessive flow represent a special kind of disability driven by both modern sensibilities and medical concerns: Variable effectiveness of menstrual hygiene products causing fears of catastrophic failure and embarrassment, the need to plan clothing and hygiene supplies around a calendar, concern that bathroom facilities might not be available if needed on short notice, and the effects of chronic hemoglobin loss, all haunt the patient with heavy menstrual flow. These drive decisions that range from accepting or declining social invitations, to the method of contraception chosen, and from traditional family treatments, to surgical interventions. It could be argued that without effective contraception, effective menstrual hygiene alternatives, and accessible therapies for heavy, painful periods, the ability of women to have open to them all options in today's society, be they career or family, would not be possible.

© Springer International Publishing AG 2018
R.P. Smith, *Dysmenorrhea and Menorrhagia*,
https://doi.org/10.1007/978-3-319-71964-1_2

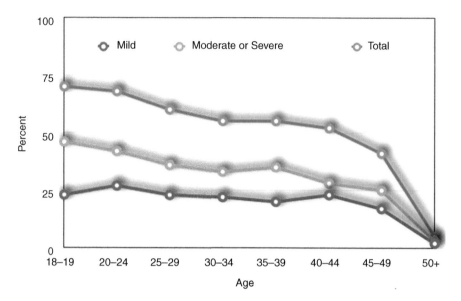

Fig. 2.1 The incidence of menstrual pain remains above 50% for women well into their 40s in a study of 934 Canadian women. Data from Burnett et al. [3]

2.2 Painful Periods

Dysmenorrhea represents the single greatest cause of lost time from work or school of any condition affecting women [4]. While it has been estimated that 30% to over 90% of the more than 75.4 million women of childbearing age in the United States (in 2012) suffer from painful menstruation, 10–20% suffer month after month discomfort sufficient to interfere with normal activities [3, 5–8]. Studies show that 70–80% of young women report having had dysmenorrhea, with almost 40% of that group reporting loss of time from school or work [3, 9]. A more recent study found almost 85% or study subjects reported feeling pain in the abdomen and back during menses [10]. Another study found that 88% of Australian women reported menstrual pain [11]. This is not a cultural or regional issue: A literature review of 50 articles showed a worldwide prevalence of some level of menstrual pain that varied from 34% (Egypt) to 94% (Oman), and the number of participants reporting very severe pain varied from 0.9% (Korea) to 59.8% (Bangladesh) [12]. Severe menstrual pain affected over 37% of 344 Saudi adolescent school girls in another report [13]. Overall, women with primary dysmenorrhea have a significantly reduced quality of life, poorer mood, and poorer sleep quality during menstruation compared with their pain-free follicular phase and compared with menses experienced by a group of pain-free control women [14] (Fig. 2.2).

Older estimates suggest that dysmenorrhea accounts for over 600 million lost working hours annually in the United States [15], but given both population growth and the ever-expanding role of women in the workforce, this number could easily

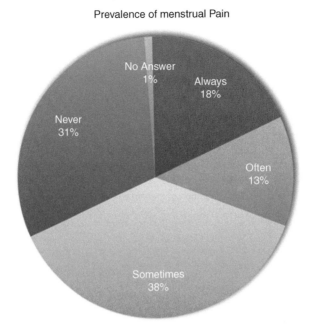

Fig. 2.2 The severity of menstrual pain as reported by 1546 Canadian women. Data from Burnett et al. [3]

underestimate the impact by as much as a factor of two. Burnett's study of Canadian women found that of those with moderate or severe pain, 51% reported that their pain had caused a limitation in their ability to function, and 24% reported missing time from school or work [3]. Indeed, in the same study, women with severe symptoms were almost ten times more likely to miss work or school as other women (37% vs. 4%). A survey of Flemish 13-year-olds found that one in four (25.4%) postmenarchal girls reported a negative impact of menstruation on social activities, but this proportion was significantly higher in girls who experienced menstruation as painful (41.3%) compared to those who did not (14.2%) [16] (Fig. 2.3).

A recent review of the adolescent dysmenorrhea found that 1/3 to 1/2 of adolescents with menstrual pain were missing school or work at least once per cycle, and more frequently in 5–14% of cases [17]. As dramatic as these statistics are, they do not consider the impact of the time lost from school and early careers by young and adolescent women—the health-related quality of life [2, 18]. Given that the peak age for dysmenorrhea occurs during the late teens and early twenties—at a time when these young women can least afford absences from their daily pursuits or education or career growth [8, 19]—the magnitude of this disability is easily understood. Some hope comes from data that supports the observation that the incidence of menstrual pain tends to gradually decline with age [20, 21], though not with parity [3]. Clearly, for most who suffers, waiting until they "outgrow" their symptoms is not an option (Fig. 2.4).

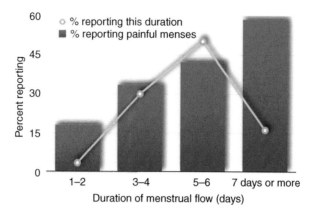

Fig. 2.3 The longer the duration of bleeding, the greater the chance of painful menses for a group of 346 Flemish girls. Data from Hoppenbrouwers et al. [16]

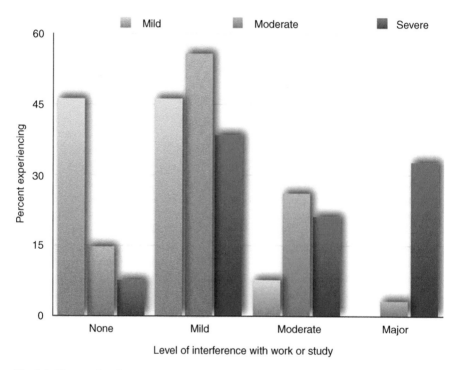

Fig. 2.4 The severity of menstrual pain directly influences the level of intrusion into work or study effectiveness. Data from Subasinghe et al. [11]

The symptoms reported by women with dysmenorrhea are many and varied. The most commonly reported manifestation of dysmenorrhea, and the one that virtually defines the condition, is crampy, midline, lower abdominal pain (often demonstrated by the patient using a fist opening and closing), which may radiate to the back or

Table 2.1 Menstrual symptoms reported in a study of students in six Mexican university programs: medicine, nursing, nutrition, dentistry, pharmacy, and psychology [6]

Symptom	Number	Percent
Cramping pain in the lower abdomen	894	93.0
Swollen abdomen	648	67.4
Irritability	480	49.9
Depression	465	48.4
Painful or tender breasts	436	45.4
Backache	414	43.1
Gastrointestinal disturbances	254	26.4
Headache	230	23.9
Swelling in the legs	178	18.5

upper thighs. In one study of 310 girls, 34% reported pain that was diffuse over the lower abdomen, suprapubic for 22.8%, in the lower back (16%), and over thighs (3.4%), with 24% of the girls reporting pain in every area [22]. Abdominal pain is closely followed in frequency by emotional symptoms, headache, syncope, and gastrointestinal disturbances such as nausea, vomiting, and diarrhea. For any given women, on any given cycle, she will often experience more than one of these. Though for each patient the pattern is generally consistent, there is still moderate variability in severity and character from month to month (Table 2.1).

Menstrual pain is a worldwide experience, but small studies indicate that the type and severity of symptoms reported can be influenced by cultural and social expectations. For example, Australian women rated menstrual pain as more intense than Chinese women, and the duration of pain was 36% longer [23]. Some studies have also suggested that women with dysmenorrhea are at greater risk for chronic pelvic pain [24]. It is not clear if this risk is related to past experience with the recurring pain of menses or if these women have a differing pain perception or threshold.

Despite continuous advances in the understanding of the pathophysiology and treatment of primary dysmenorrhea, many patients continue to suffer disability, most often because they are unaware of, or do not seek out, effective options. Some authors report that only 14–20% of young women with primary dysmenorrhea receive prescription pain treatments [4, 8, 25] even when the pain is routinely moderate or severe [3], and less than 50% seek any professional care [3]. These women often turn to over-the-counter therapies that offer variable amounts of relief [26]. In one study, almost all (98%) of adolescents used non-pharmacologic methods such as heat, rest, or distraction to treat dysmenorrhea but achieved effectiveness of 40% or less [27]. In other studies, 30–70% of girls reported at least occasionally self-medicating with over-the-counter pain medications [5, 28]. However, 57% of those who self-medicated with these preparations used sub-therapeutic doses [28], and only 54% of adolescents knew that certain medications could relieve menstrual cramps [29]. Twenty-seven percent of respondents could not recognize any of three nonsteroidal anti-inflammatory drugs (NSAID) offered as possible effective treatments for dysmenorrhea [8]. Even when adolescents seek care, they frequently are not offered any treatments [8] (Fig. 2.5).

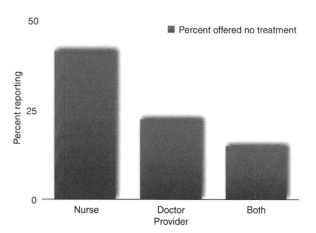

Fig. 2.5 The percentage of adolescents who were not offered care for their dysmenorrhea symptoms. Data from Hillen et al. [8]

Studies indicate that 95% of adolescent girls have taken acetaminophen either singly or in combination with other over-the-counter medications for relief of dysmenorrhea [28]—a strategy that often results in undertreatment and persistent symptoms. Small projects have reported that simple educational interventions can significantly improve appropriate treatment, resulting in symptom reduction [30]. Therefore, education, either of individuals or of groups, is an investment well worth making for these women.

2.3   Heavy Periods

There has long been an association between painful and heavy menstrual periods [16]. In one study, bleeding duration was found to be significantly associated with dysmenorrhea, and girls with bleeding duration more than 5 days had an almost twofold increase in the risk of pain. Moreover, girls with the presence of clots had more than twice as much chance of having dysmenorrhea [22]. Like dysmenorrhea, heavy menstrual bleeding is common among adolescent and young women, with prevalence rates that exceed 30% [31–33] (Fig. 2.6).

Heavy menstrual bleeding (menorrhagia) is defined as menstrual blood loss >80 mL per cycle [34]. This value was derived from work that showed that anemia was common when blood loss exceeds this level. Because it is difficult to objectively evaluate menstrual blood loss [35], heavy menstrual bleeding is also functionally defined as excessive menstrual blood loss that interferes with the woman's physical, emotional, social, and material quality of life, and can occur alone or in combination with other symptoms [36]. Historical clinical indicators of heavy flow have been the number of pads or tampons used, the frequency of changes, the use of double protection (both pad and tampon), the degree of soiling, and the presence or absence of clots. Regrettably, the reliability to predict actual blood loss with these observations has been poor [37–39]. Despite these limitations, several aspects of

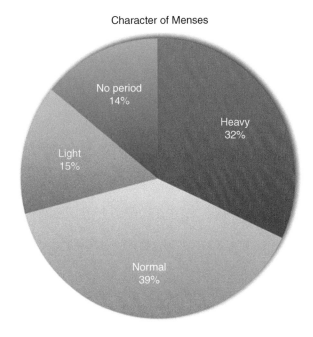

Character of Menses

Fig. 2.6 The character of menstrual flow for 1547 women, aged 40–45 years old in Sweden. Data from Karlsson et al. [31]

Table 2.2 Perceptions surrounding menstruation reported by 1547 women, aged 40–45 years old with heavy and normal menstrual flow

Perception	Those with heavy flow (%)	Those with normal flow (%)
Bleeding is awkward	92	78
I get less done	62	37
I feel out of sorts	79	65
I feel feminine	34	40
I feel unclean	90	83

All differences were statistically significant at $p < 0.001$ except for "I feel feminine." Data from Karlsson et al. [31]

these menstrual characteristics have been adopted for such things as pictorial guides [40] and online assessment tools [41].

Like menstrual pain, heavy menstrual bleeding can represent an intrusive disruption for young women, affecting their functionality and self-image [31]. These women consistently report associated fatigue, lethargy, and problems concentrating. In a study involving high school students, there was a strong correlation between the amount of bleeding and the negative impact on quality of life [42]. An investigation of 48 adolescent girls with heavy menstrual bleeding compared to 102 controls found that 79.2% with heavy menstrual bleeding reported that their bleeding affected their ability to participate in physical education class or sports, versus only 36.3% of the controls [43] (Table 2.2).

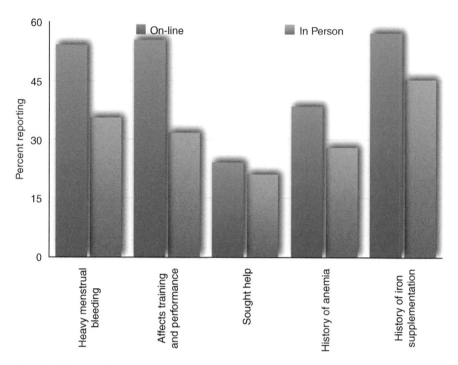

Fig. 2.7 Characteristics of menses as experienced by a group of amateur athletes. Data from Bruinvels et al. [45]

Menstruation is the most common single cause of iron deficiency anemia in women of childbearing age [44]. In an online and in-person survey of women marathon participants (789 participants online and 1073 in-person interviews at the race), heavy menstrual bleeding was reported by 54% of the online group and by 36% of the in-person marathon runners. Overall, 32% of these active women reported a history of anemia, and 50% had previously supplemented with iron [45]. This level of anemia requiring supplementation is less than was found (63%) in a recent Europe-wide study a diagnosis of heavy menstrual bleeding [46]. Despite the athlete's self-acknowledged heavy flow, only a minority (22%) had sought medical advice [45]. It is likely that the increased body awareness of these runners may explain a greater wiliness to seek help compared to the general population that seek help at rates as low as 6% [47] (Fig. 2.7).

Because of the inability to accurately quantify menstrual blood loss in the clinical setting and the absence of simple diagnostic or therapeutic options, surgical therapy is often the easy choice. In one review, a referral to an attending gynecologist for heavy menstrual bleeding meant a 43% chance of a hysterectomy [48] and a 75% 5-year risk of surgery [49]. Heavy menstrual bleeding is the major justification for the approximately 300,000 hysterectomies performed yearly in the United States [50].

Key Points
- Both menstrual pain and heavy menstrual bleeding are common sources of disability for adolescent and young women.
- Menstrual pain and heavy menstrual flow are found together.
- Dysmenorrhea in young patients often goes undiagnosed and undertreated.
- When self-medication is used for menstrual symptoms, relief is generally poor.
- Accurate assessment of the quantity of menstrual loss is very difficult in the clinical setting.

References

1. Collett B. Visceral pain: the importance of pain management services. Br J Pain. 2013;7(1):6–7.
2. Nur Azurah AG, Sanci L, Moore E, Grover S. The quality of life of adolescents with menstrual problems. J Pediatr Adolesc Gynecol. 2013;26(2):102–8.
3. Burnett MA, Antao V, Black A, et al. Prevalence of primary dysmenorrhea in Canada. J Obstet Gynaecol Can. 2005;27:765–70.
4. Klein JR, Litt IF. Epidemiology of adolescent dysmenorrhea. Pediatrics. 1981;68:661–4.
5. Andersch B, Milson I. An epidemiologic study of young women with dysmenorrhea. Am J Obstet Gynecol. 1982;144:655–60.
6. Ortiz MI. Primary dysmenorrhea among Mexican university students: prevalence, impact and treatment. Eur J Obstet Gynecol Reprod Biol. 2010;152:73–7.
7. Polat A, Celik H, Gurates B, et al. Prevalence of primary dysmenorrhea in young adult female university students. Arch Gynecol Obstet. 2009;279:527–32.
8. Hillen TI, Grbavac SL, Johnston PJ, et al. Primary dysmenorrhea in young Western Australian women: prevalence, impact, and knowledge of treatment. J Adolesc Health. 1999;25:40–5.
9. Agarwal A, Venkat A. Questionnaire study on menstrual disorders in adolescent girls in Singapore. J Pediatr Adolesc Gynecol. 2009;22:365–71.
10. Kamel DM, Tantawy SA, Abdelsamea GA. Experience of dysmenorrhea among a group of physical therapy students from Cairo University: an exploratory study. J Pain Res. 2017;10:1079–85.
11. Subasinghe AK, Happo L, Jayasinghe YL, Garland SM, Gorelik A, Wark JD. Prevalence and severity of dysmenorrhoea, and management options reported by young Australian women. Aust Fam Physician. 2016;45(11):829–34.
12. De Sanctis V, Soliman AT, Elsedfy H, Soliman NA, Soliman R, El Kholy M. Dysmenorrhea in adolescents and young adults: a review in different country. Acta Biomed. 2017;87(3):233–46.
13. Abd El-Mawgod MM, Alshaibany AS, Al-Anazi AM. Epidemiology of dysmenorrhea among secondary-school students in Northern Saudi Arabia. J Egypt Public Health Assoc. 2016;91(3):115–9.
14. Iacovides S, Avidon I, Baker FC. What we know about primary dysmenorrhea today: a critical review. Hum Reprod Update. 2015;21(6):762–78.
15. Smith RP. Gynecology in primary care. Baltimore, MD: Williams and Wilkins; 1996. p. 471–500.
16. Hoppenbrouwers K, Roelants M, Meuleman C, et al. Characteristics of the menstrual cycle in 13-year-old Flemish girls and the impact of menstrual symptoms on social life. Eur J Pediatr. 2016;175(5):623–30.
17. De Sanctis V, Soliman A, Bernasconi S, et al. Primary dysmenorrhea in adolescents: prevalence, impact and recent knowledge. Pediatr Endocrinol Rev. 2015;13(2):512–20.
18. Grandi G, Ferrari S, Xholli A, et al. Prevalence of menstrual pain in young women: what is dysmenorrhea? J Pain Res. 2012;5:169–74.

19. Svanborg L, Ulmsten U. The incidence of primary dysmenorrhea in teenagers. Arch Gynecol. 1981;230:173–7.
20. Sundell G, Milsom I, Andersch B. Factors influencing the prevalence and severity of dysmenorrhoea in young women. Br J Obstet Gynaecol. 1990;97:588–94.
21. Weissman AM, Hartz AJ, Hansen MD, Johnson SR. The natural history of primary dysmenorrhea: a longitudinal study. BJOG. 2004;111:345–52.
22. Kural M, Noor NN, Pandit D, Joshi T, Patil A. Menstrual characteristics and prevalence of dysmenorrhea in college going girls. J Family Med Prim Care. 2015;4(3):426–31.
23. Zhu X, Wong F, Bensoussan A, Lo SK, Zhou C, Yu J. Are there any cross-ethnic differences in menstrual profiles? A pilot comparative study on Australian and Chinese women with primary dysmenorrhea. J Obstet Gynaecol Res. 2010;36(5):1093–101.
24. Westling AM, Tu FF, Griffith JW, Hellman KM. The association of dysmenorrhea with noncyclic pelvic pain accounting for psychological factors. Am J Obstet Gynecol. 2013;209(5):422. e1–10.
25. Wildholm O. Dysmenorrhea during adolescence. Acta Obstet Gynaecol Scand. 1979;87(Suppl):61–6.
26. Zhang WY, Li Wan Po A. Efficacy of minor analgesics in primary dysmenorrhoea: a systematic review. Br J Obstet Gynaecol. 1998;105:780–9.
27. Campbell MA, McGrath PJ. Non-pharmacologic strategies used by adolescents for the management of menstrual discomfort. Clin J Pain. 1999;15:313–20.
28. Campbell MA, McGrath PJ. Use of medication by adolescents for the management of menstrual discomfort. Arch Pediatr Adolesc Med. 1997;151:905–13.
29. Johnson J. Level of knowledge among adolescent girls regarding effective treatment for dysmenorrhea. J Adolesc Health. 1988;9:398–402.
30. Jung HS, Lee J. Prevalence of primary dysmenorrhea in young adult female university students. Eur J Obstet Gynecol Reprod Biol. 2013;170(2):480–6.
31. Karlsson TS, Marions LB, Edlund MG. Heavy menstrual bleeding significantly affects quality of life. Acta Obstet Gynecol Scand. 2014;93:52–7.
32. Santos IS, Minten GC, Valle NC, et al. Menstrual bleeding patterns: a community-based cross-sectional study among women aged 18–45 years in Southern Brazil. BMC Womens Health. 2011;11:26–33.
33. Friberg B, Ornö AK, Lindgren A, Lethagen S. Bleeding disorders among young women: a population-based prevalence study. Acta Obstet Gynecol Scand. 2006;85:200–6.
34. Hallberg L, Hogdahl AM, Nilsson L, Rybo G. Menstrual blood loss – a population study. Acta Obstet Gynaecol Scand. 1966;45:320–51.
35. Chimbira TH, Anderson ABM, Turnbull AC. Relation between measured menstrual loss and the patient's subjective assessment of loss, duration of bleeding, numbers of sanitary towels used, uterine weight and endometrial surface area. Br J Obstet Gynaecol. 1980;87:603–8.
36. Munro MG, Critchley HO, Fraser IS. The FIGO systems for nomenclature and classification of causes of abnormal uterine bleeding in the reproductive years: who needs them? Am J Obstet Gynecol. 2012;207:259–65.
37. Haynes PJ, Hodgson H, Anderson ABM, Turnbull AC. Measurement of menstrual blood loss in patients complaining of menorrhagia. Br J Obstet Gynaecol. 1977;84:763–8.
38. Fraser IS, MaCarron G, Markham R, Resta T. Blood and total fluid content of menstrual discharge. Obstet Gynecol. 1985;65:194–8.
39. Schumacher U, Schumacher J, Mellinger U, Gerlinger C, Wienke A, Endrikat J. Estimation of menstrual blood loss volume based on menstrual diary and laboratory data. BMC Womens Health. 2012;12:24–31.
40. Higham JM, O'Brien PM, Shaw RM. Assessment of menstrual blood loss using a pictorial chart. Br J Obstet Gynaecol. 1990;8:734–9.
41. Grabell J, Albert S, Young J, et al. Generation and optimization of the self-administered bleeding assessment tool and its validation as a screening test for von Willebrand disease. Haemophilia. 2015;21(5):e384–8.

42. Pawar A, Krishnan R, Davis K, Bosma K, Kulkarni R. Perceptions about quality of life in a school-based population of adolescents with menorrhagia: implications for adolescents with bleeding disorders. Haemophilia. 2008;14:579–83.
43. Wang W, Bourgeois T, Klima J, Berlan ED, Fischer AN, O'Brien SH. Iron deficiency and fatigue in adolescent females with heavy menstrual bleeding. Haemophilia. 2013;19:225–30.
44. Taylor S, Rampton D. Treatment of iron deficiency anemia: practical considerations. Pol Arch Med Wewn. 2015;125:452–60.
45. Bruinvels G, Burden R, Brown N, Richards T, Pedlar C. The prevalence and impact of heavy menstrual bleeding (menorrhagia) in elite and non-elite athletes. PLoS One. 2016;11(2):e0149881.
46. Fraser IS, Mansour D, Breymann C, Hoffman C, Mezzacasa A, Petraglia F. Prevalence of heavy menstrual bleeding and experiences of affected women in a European patient survey. Int J Gynaecol Obstet. 2015;128:196–200.
47. McCormick A, Fleming D, Charlton J. Morbidity statistics from general practice: fourth national study 1991–1992. London: HMSO; 1995.
48. Coulter A, Bradlow J, Agass M, Martin-Bates C, Tulloch A. Outcomes of referrals to gynaecology outpatient clinics for menstrual problems: an audit of general practice records. Br J Obstet Gynaecol. 1991;98:789–96.
49. Royal College of Obstetricians and Gynaecologists. RCOG evidence-based clinical guideline number 1: the initial management of menorrhagia. London: RCOG; 1998.
50. James AH, Ragni MV, Picozzi VJ. Bleeding disorders in premenopausal women: (another) public health crisis for hematology? Hematology Am Soc Hematol Educ Program. 2006;2006:474–85.

Additional Resources

A general review:
Davies J, Kadir RA. Heavy menstrual bleeding: an update on management. Thromb Res. 2017;151(Suppl 1):S70–7.
Practice Bulletins from the American College of Obstetricians and Gynecologists:
American College of Obstetricians and Gynecologists. Diagnosis of abnormal uterine bleeding in reproductive-aged women. Practice Bulletin No. 128. Obstet Gynecol. 2012;120:197–206.
American College of Obstetricians and Gynecologists. Noncontraceptive uses of hormonal contraceptives. Practice Bulletin No. 110. Obstet Gynecol. 2010;115:206–18.
An excellent compilation of studies:
National Collaborating Centre for Women's and Children's Health (UK). Heavy menstrual bleeding. London: RCOG Press; 2007. January (NICE Clinical Guidelines, No. 44).

Chapter 3
How Our Views Have Evolved: Historical Perspectives

3.1 Overview

Menstruation has been treated as everything from an ordinary event to evidence of a "curse." Menstruating women have been treated as unclean, shunned, exiled, or ridiculed. It was well known that the touch of a menstruating woman would cause baking bread to fall, flowers to wilt, and brass to tarnish. During her period, a Muslim woman is not allowed inside a Mosque and cannot pray or fast during Ramadan. Even the Bible notes that whenever a woman has her menstrual period, she and those who touch her are "ceremonially unclean" for up to 7 days (Leviticus 15:19–33). This is their lot to deal with, preferably well away from the eyes of a male-dominated society. (The word "taboo" itself comes from the Polynesian word *tapua* which means "menstruation.") When strong opiate analgesics failed to control the pain of menstrual cramps, it was easier to attribute the disability to being "all in the head" than to admit to a lack of understanding about the underlying pathophysiology. Ironically, some of these vary myths have led to today's understanding of dysmenorrhea and menorrhagia and have made it possible for us to talk about prevention rather than relief. Indeed, the success of moving from symptoms to pathophysiology, from amelioration to prevention in dysmenorrhea, paved the way for similar efforts in conditions ranging from interstitial cystitis to migraine headaches. Understanding that journey provides valuable perspectives when we deal with patients who still suffer from these conditions.

3.2 Menstruation and Menstrual Hygiene

Any discussion of menstrual hygiene or dysfunction prior to written records would be complete speculation, though there is no reason to believe that menstrual pain or a complete spectrum of menstrual blood loss from light to heavy would not have existed from the time of our hominid progenitors. (It should be noted that regular menstrual cycle is predicated on the overall health and nutrition of the woman, so

© Springer International Publishing AG 2018
R.P. Smith, *Dysmenorrhea and Menorrhagia*,
https://doi.org/10.1007/978-3-319-71964-1_3

that regular monthly cycles are likely a (relatively) more modern phenomenon.) While there are records in Egyptian hieroglyphics suggesting the use of intravaginal items to prevent conception, there is no definitive evidence for tampons or other items for menstrual hygiene, despite occasional tampon advertising to the contrary (An inscription at the Hathor temple in Edfu does contain a list of gods with their specific dislikes, including one that disliked menstruating women [1] (Fig. 3.1).)

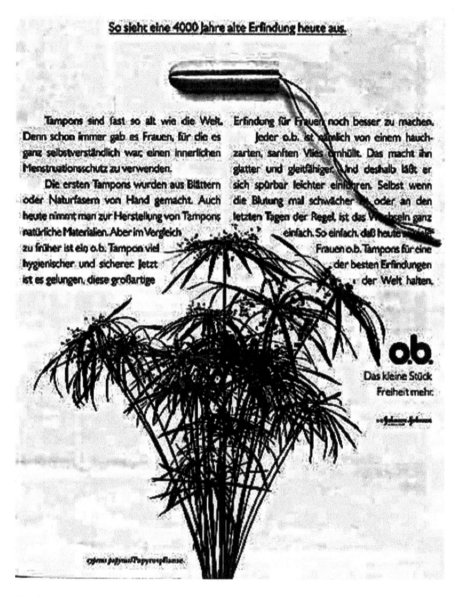

Fig. 3.1 An advertisement for o.b. tampons from the German magazine Burda (1989) claiming a historic link to Egyptian papyrus tampons

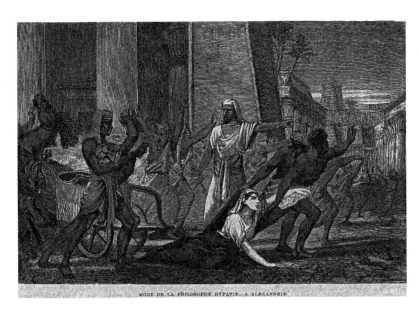

MORT DE LA PHILOSOPHE HYPATIE. A ALEXANDRIE.

Fig. 3.2 "Death of the philosopher Hypatia, in Alexandria" from *Vies des savants illustres, depuis l'antiquité jusqu'au dix-neuvième siècle*, 1866, by Louis Figuier. Many historians view the murder of Hypatia as the end of Classical antiquity

While the historic (pre-twentieth century) heritage for menstrual tampons is almost impossible to establish, the use of perineal pads for menstrual hygiene is better documented [2]. Roman women used absorbent cotton pads and linen underwear (*subligaculum*). Hypatia of Alexandria (c. 350–370 to 415 CE), the Greek mathematician, astronomer, and philosopher in Egypt, then a part of the Eastern Roman Empire, is reported to have used menstrual pads (*pannus menstruus,* translated from a Greek term, "the rhakoi of women"—Rhakoi are "rags") (Fig. 3.2).

Except for the fashionable ladies of sixteenth-century Italy, between the medieval era and the early 1800s, most women (and men) did not wear undergarments. In medieval Europe, women carried nosegays of sweet-smelling herbs around their necks and waists, in the hopes of neutralizing the odor of blood, though the general lack of bathing suggests additional advantages as well.

In the absence of undergarments, if menstrual pads were worn, they would have been held in place with belts or girdles. For example, Queen Elizabeth I of England (1558–1603) is known to have owned three black silk girdles to keep in place her linen sanitary towels or *vallopes of Holland cloth* [3, 4]—Holland cloth is a plain-woven or dull-finish linen, but the term often just referred to any linens imported from Europe, particularly from the Netherlands. (These must have been at least somewhat effective because there are contemporary reports that court watchers of the period speculated that the queen never menstruated, going so far as to try to bribe the royal laundresses for information [5].) Even today, in less-developed countries, menstrual cloths are still looped over a string around the waist in the absence of undergarments (Fig. 3.3).

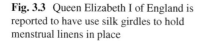
Fig. 3.3 Queen Elizabeth I of England is reported to have use silk girdles to hold menstrual linens in place

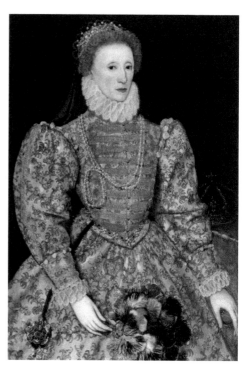

When underwear did return to use, for women it often had an open crotch to allow for bodily functions and to avoid soiling from ineffective and leaking menstrual hygiene efforts. To augment clothing protection, women frequently wore a sanitary apron, hanging toward the back, that protected the back of her garments. In England, Southalls of Birmingham advertised disposable menstrual pads in 1888, suitable for "Ladies Travelling by Land and Sea," and Lister's Towels, created by Johnson & Johnson, where marketed in the United States beginning in 1896. But because the morality of the time prevented advertising these "unmentionables," the product did not reach many women and was eventually withdrawn from the market, though the name continued to be seen in print advertising into the late 1920s (Figs. 3.4 and 3.5).

It wasn't until after World War I that truly absorbent menstrual pads became widely available, when the leftover cellucotton (wood pulp fiber) from the field bandages of the war's aid stations provided the inspiration for the development and marketing of what became Kotex brand sanitary pads. Despite wide distribution, sales were slow until Montgomery Ward advertised them in their catalog, and the packaging was changed to a discrete blue with little to identify the product (Fig. 3.6).

Despite the debate about the historical origins of menstrual tampons, it was only in 1933 that the modern applicator-style tampon was patented (US Pat # 1,926,900, September 12, 1933). Acceptance by women was slow, and there was even strong

Fig. 3.4 A 1914 US Patent
for a sanitary apron
granted to Leah Milken

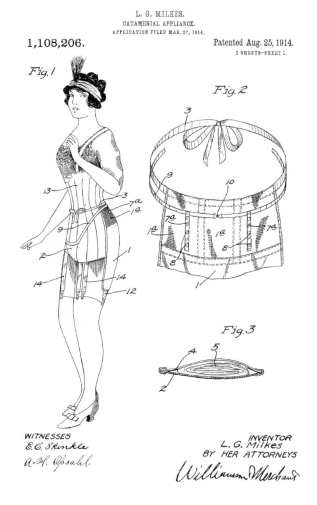

Fig. 3.5 An early shop
sign for Lister's Towels (c.
1907–9)

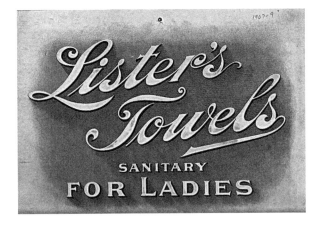

Fig. 3.6 Ad copy from a 1921 magazine advertisement for Kotex sanitary pads emphasizing the tie to war-time bandages that were their origins

NEW but tried and proved, Kotex enters universal service from a romantic background. For, although a woman's article, it started as Cellucotton — a wonderful sanitary absorbent which science perfected for use of our men and allied soldiers wounded in France.

With peace came an idea suggested in letters from nurses in France, regarding a new use for this wonderful absorbent, and early in 1919 our laboratory made the first sanitary pads of Cellucotton enclosed in gauze and placed them on sale in various cities. Requests for more followed every sale, and we devoted two years to perfecting the new article—named KOTEX from "cotton-like texture"—and to the building of machinery which makes and seals it hygienically without contact of human hands. Kotex are now ready for every woman's use.

The gauze envelope is 22 inches long, thus leaving generous tabs for pinning. The filler, thirty-six layers of finest Cellucotton, is 3½ inches wide by 9 inches long. Kotex are cool, more absorbent, and of lasting softness. Kotex are cheap in price and easy to throw away.

CELLUCOTTON PRODUCTS CO.
208 South LaSalle Street, Chicago, Illinois

resistance by some in the medical community because of issues of virginity and the need to touch the vulva. Even as late as 1945, an article in *The Journal of the American Medical Association* still had to include nine illustrations of how tampons worked, how they should be worn, and why they provided a more sanitary option to perineal pads [6] (Fig. 3.7).

3.3   Understanding Physiology

The Ebers Papyrus (c. 1552 BCE) portrayed the uterus as a wandering animal, usually a tortoise, newt, or crocodile, capable of movement within its host. Inflammations, excitations, and malpositions also ruled as the causes of female complaints [7]. Supporting this philosophy was Aretaeus, a physician from Cappadocia, who was a contemporary of Galen. In the second century CE, he wrote that the uterus could move out of place, and float within the body, "like an animal within an animal." If it moved up, it could cause sluggishness, weakness, and vertigo. Should it descend, there would be a strong sense of choking, loss of speech and sensibility, and, most ominously, the possibility of sudden death (Fig. 3.8).

During the middle ages, medical thought was dominated by religious convictions, belief in a limited number of experts, and preoccupation with war, plague, and other more pressing issues. This was when the seven-cell doctrine of uterine structure emerged, replacing the animalistic concept of a wandering parasite. This new anatomic view depicted the uterine cavity as divided into seven compartments with male embryos developing on the right, female on the left, and hermaphrodites in the center [8]. This idea may have arisen because of the influence of the *De spermate, Microtegni, and De XII portis*, a pseudo-Galenic treatise used from the twelfth century, which claimed that most parts of the body were divided into sevens [9], corresponding with the days of the week. This composite structural view

Fig. 3.7 The illustration that accompanied US Patent number 1,926,900 (issued September 12, 1933) for the first commercially made tampon for menstrual hygiene

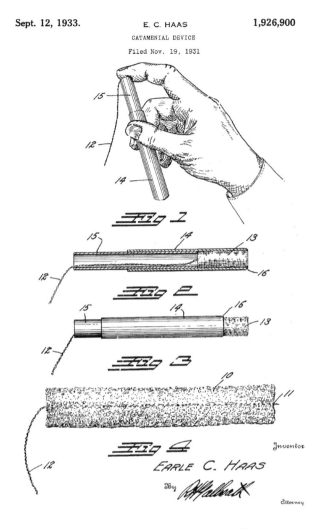

Sept. 12, 1933.

E. C. HAAS

1,926,900

CATAMENIAL DEVICE

Filed Nov. 19, 1931

of the uterus firmly anchored the organ to the pelvis, but the complex functions of the uterus, beyond as a pregnancy vessel, remained unknown (Fig. 3.9).

In the west, even the connection between ovulation and menstruation was not made until about 1821, when John Power discussed the possibility in his *Essays on the Female Economy* [10]. The connection was not fully adopted until 1831, with the writings of Charles Négrier reporting his autopsy studies [11–14]. While the Dutch anatomist Reinier de Graaf first described the follicle in 1668, even the idea that the follicle did not represent the ovum itself wasn't recognized until 1827, by Karl Ernst von Baer [15] (Figs. 3.10 and 3.11).

As the understanding of the physiology of menstruation matured, so did the perception that menstruation and its dysfunction were natural processes and not one driven by divine retribution, superstition, or mystery. This opened the opportunity to view the extremes of the menstrual experience (pain, heavy and light periods, etc.) as pathologies that could be studied, explained, and treated. Without that full

Fig. 3.8 The Ebers
Papyrus details many of
the views of women's
health held in ancient
Egypt

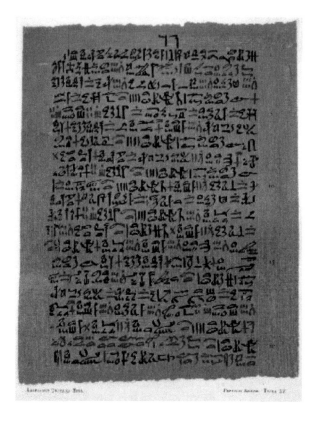

Fig. 3.9 An illustration of
the seven chambers of the
uterus

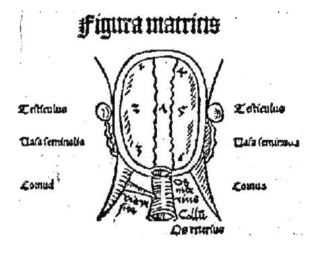

Fig. 3.10 The Dutch
anatomist, Reinier de
Graaf (July 30, 1641–
August 17, 1673), for
whom the Graafian follicle
is named

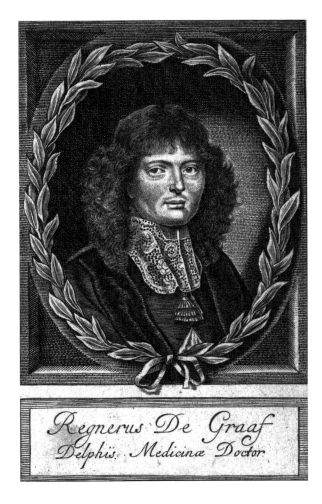

Fig. 3.11 The ovary as
rendered by Reinier de
Graaf

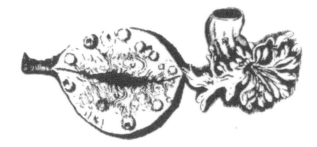

understanding, even into the twentieth century, treatments such as cautery of the middle turbinate of the nose for menstrual pain [16] could be found. The roots of this new appreciation for the physiology of the uterus were first set down during our earliest prehistory with the identification of those affected.

3.4 Recognition of Dysfunction

The word "dysmenorrhea" is derived from a Greek root meaning difficult monthly flow, but did not make its appearance in the English language until about 1810 [17]. Despite the late arrival of our current term, menstrual pain has almost certainly been a part of women's lot for millennia—Catholic doctrine goes so far as to allege that the pain of childbirth and menstruation is a retribution for Eve's betrayal of God's trust in the Garden of Eden, even though it was Adam who ate the forbidden fruit from the Tree of Knowledge (Fig. 3.12).

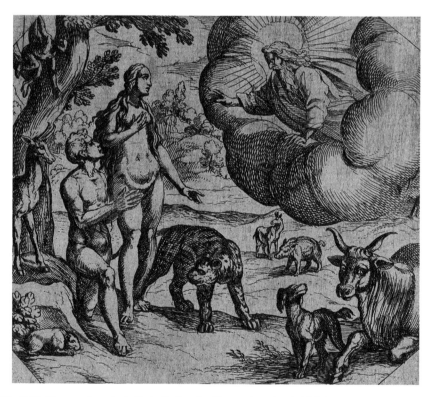

Fig. 3.12 Eve was the culprit. Catholic doctrine blames the pain of childbirth and menstruation on Eve's role in mankind's expulsion from God's grace and the Garden of Eden (Image: Los Angeles County Museum of Art, www.lacma.org)

The recognition that menstruation can be associated with dysfunction has been documented for almost as long as written records exist. The Kahun Gynecological Papyrus, dated to about 1800 BCE, contains references to pain in the womb and suggests specific treatments to be applied [18]. Later writings, including the Ebers Papyrus, include prescriptions for fenugreek and complex potions that were used by Egyptian women to ease menstrual pain. Pliny reported the use of bitumen for symptoms of congestion of the womb and prolapse [19]. In China, agents such as dong quai came into favor for their effectiveness in relieving menstrual pain. In Australia, aboriginal people used a decoction of raspberry leaves as a traditional treatment for painful menstruation, childbirth, flu, and morning sickness [20] (Fig. 3.13).

The *Hippocratic Corpus*, a compilation of works written by various authors between the fifth and fourth centuries BCE, describes menorrhagia as a potential cause for illness [21], rather than a pathology itself, proclaiming "When the menses are excessive, diseases take place" [22]. Heavy flow was also associated with "grumulous clots... accompanied with pain, inflammation of the uterus, [and] hysteric paroxysms," acknowledging the link between heavy flow and menstrual pain.

The Greek physician, Pedanius Dioscorides (40–90 CE), in his *De Materia Medica* (the precursor to all modern pharmacopeias, written about 50–70 CE), recognized menstrual pain as an organic, pathologic condition requiring treatment and recommending several multipart mixtures and treatments [23]. This treatise influenced medical thought and practice well into the middle ages. Soranus of Ephesus (98–138 CE), the Greek physician, advocated the application of a bladder filled with hot oil and held over the lower abdomen to treat menstrual pain [24], foreshadowing today's renewed interest in topical heat therapy (Fig. 3.14).

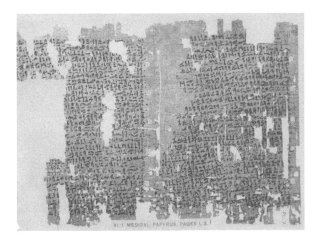

Fig. 3.13 Page 1 and part of page 2 of the Kahun Gynecological Papyrus, c. 1800 BCE

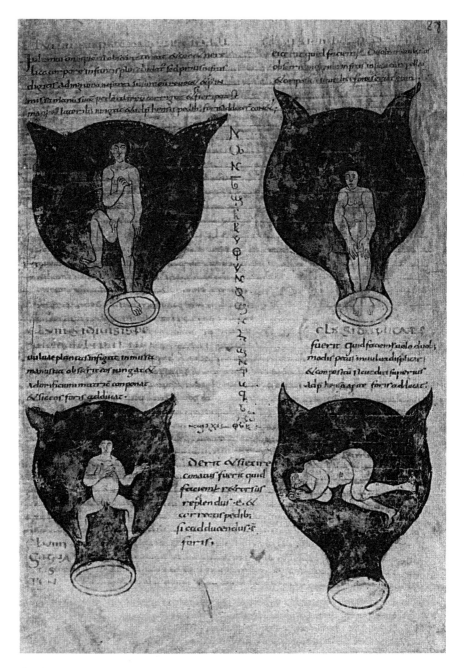

Fig. 3.14 Soranus of Ephesus (98–138 CE) wrote extensively on medicine and the ailments of women. Shown here are illustrations of the positions of the fetus in the uterus. (Soranus of Ephesus, gynecology, in a Latin version of Late Antiquity: positions of the embryo in the uterus. The illustrations in this medieval manuscript are probably based on drawings by Soranus. Brussels, Bibliothèque Royale, Codex 3714, fol. 28r)

Fig. 3.15 Mass marketed from 1876 on, *Lydia E. Pinkham's Vegetable Compound* became one of the best-known patent medicines of the nineteenth century

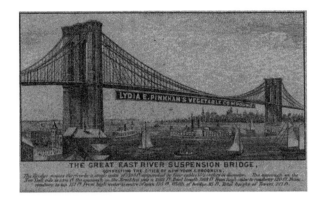

Paulus of Aegina (c. 625–c.690 CE) advocated using ligatures applied to the armpits and groins to reduce blood flow to the body and, thus, to the uterus [25]. In the traditional Unani system of medicine, dry cupping therapy (hijamat bila shurt) has been used to treat menorrhagia [26], something that had even been advocated by Hippocrates. Even saffron has been prescribed for menstrual pain and heavy flow, continuing a tradition of herbal treatments that reached its height in the widely popular herbal-alcoholic "women's tonic," *Lydia Pinkham's Vegetable Compound*, which is still available (in altered formulation) even today. (Lydia Pinkham is credited by some as the first successful American businesswoman, due to the great success of this patent medicine (Fig. 3.15).)

Western medicine made remarkable strides in the understanding of anatomy and physiology, including extensive writings on menstruation and its abnormalities, during the 1800s [27]. Despite this body of science, even into the last century, many viewed menstrual pain as "like headache, is an expression of discomfort, not a disease nor a pathologic entity" [28]. This did not stop the introduction of myriad alcoholic and narcotic concoctions that were marketed for "women's complaints." These were common until the 1906 Pure Food and Drug Act, signed by President Theodore Roosevelt, that required disclosure of the ingredients contained in consumer products and led to the creation of the Food and Drug Administration. Under the law, drug labels had to disclose any of ten ingredients that were deemed "addictive" and/or "dangerous," if they were present, and could not list them if they were not present. Alcohol, morphine, opium (laudanum), and cannabis were all included on the list, leading to the withdrawal of many of the products women had come to rely on (Fig. 3.16).

Given that the written knowledge we have of ancient cultures was exclusively written by men, the acknowledgment of pain or heavy bleeding reflects the magnitude of the associated disability. Without the foundational acceptance of the existence of pathology and the related physiology, truly effective treatments could not become available.

Fig. 3.16 An early twentieth-century advertisement for "Hall's Coca Wine," one of many cocaine-laced tonics touted for a range of conditions including "sickness, so common to ladies," a euphemism for menstruation and its associated pain. (Image: Wellcome Library, London. Wellcome Images)

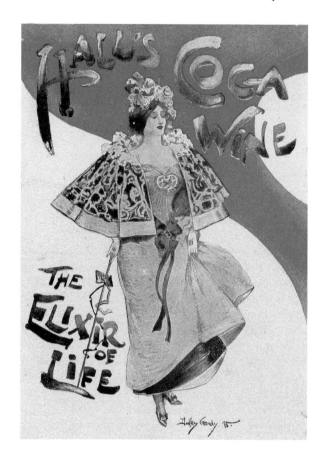

3.5   The Causes of Menstrual Dysfunction

Many nineteenth-century textbook writers (e.g., Thomas, [29]) classified menstrual pain into neuralgic, congestive, inflammatory, obstructive, and membranous types, based primarily on the symptoms reported. Others attributed menstrual pain to atrophy or an immature uterus, suggesting that marriage or childbirth would provide relief. For this immaturity, "exercise" by the placement of a stem pessary (an intracervical device), which would cause the uterus to contract to attempt to expel the device, was advised [30]. Regular pelvic massage or intercourse was recommended to "open the uterus." This treatment was recommended for everything from hysteria to menstrual cramps, leading to the introduction (in 1883) and acceptance of "medical" massagers, that today we would recognize as "vibrators." (These treatments were considered most effective if "hysterical paroxysms"—orgasms—occurred (Fig. 3.17).)

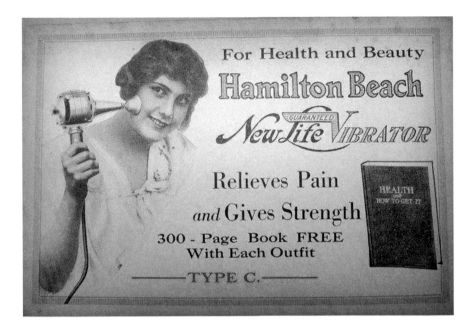

Fig. 3.17 Companies such as A.C. Gilbert, Co. and Hamilton Beach had been making medical vibrators since the late 1800s. Later they began making home versions of the medical vibrators, like this 1912 model. These large units, powered by plugging into electrical power, reached their peak popularity in the 1920s and 1930s, gradually being replaced by smaller, lighter, more discrete battery-powered devices

Later classifications of menstrual pain focused upon the causes of pain, rather than the symptoms, tacitly recognizing the condition as a pathology. These schemas acknowledged that the possible etiologies for menstrual abnormalities encountered could arise either from the uterus itself or from conditions acquired or "extrinsic" to it [31, 32]. Because of an incomplete understanding of the physiology underlying much of the reproductive organs and cycle, it was common to attribute dysfunction to malformation, malposition, or to simply write off the symptoms as psychogenic. Just as with the notion of the "wandering uterus" as the cause of hysteria, malposition of the uterus was seen as the cause of all manner of complaints (Fig. 3.18).

3.6 Uterine Activity Studies

The first successful attempts to measure uterine activity occurred in 1872 [34, 35] and predate the development of the sphygmomanometer [36], though little use was made of the technology at the time. Following Rucker's 1925 report of uterine activity in a nonpregnant woman [37], a new interest in uterine physiology outside of pregnancy was spurred. Increased uterine contractions were hypothesized as a cause

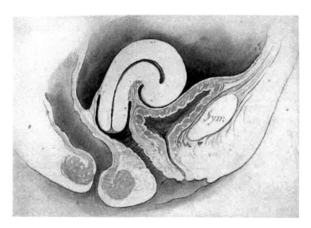

Fig. 3.18 "Congenital anteflexion of the uterus, the chief lesion in patients with congenital dysmenorrhea. The cervix is usually long, the canal tight, the fundus sharply flexed" [33]

of dysmenorrhea in 1932 [38], and by the late 1930s, objective findings began to support the concept of a physical (uterine) cause for the symptoms reported. Though large amplitude contractions were found in one study of 11 dysmenorrheic women [39], the extreme interest in the effects of newly discovered hormones at the time diverted the attention of investigators in that direction, diminishing the impact of these findings.

The relationship between uterine activity and menstrual pain was bolstered by studies of simultaneous electrical and mechanical changes carried out by Jacobsen and Lackner, in 1939 and 1940 [40, 41]. Using an intrauterine air-filled balloon system, Wilson and Kurzrok also noted the relationship of maximal uterine activity and pain [42, 43]. Despite these studies, little change occurred in the way dysmenorrhea was viewed or was treated—the tools to take advantage of this information simply did not exist.

By the late 1940s, it was finally accepted that women with dysmenorrhea had fundamental differences in the mechanical activity of their uterus. Liessé, in France, showed that these women also had more electrical and mechanical activity that directly correlated with the pain of menstruation [44]. He found irregular electrical discharges of as much as 30 per second during pain, with minimal activity occurring between pains. These studies suggested a cause (electrical) for dysmenorrhea but could provide no clue to the underlying disturbance in physiology that resulted in the observed discharges.

The most detailed and influential studies of dysmenorrhea and uterine activity came in 1947, in work by Woodbury [45]. His findings of direct correlations between pressure, pattern of contractions, resting tone, and pain became a standard reference. While these findings were verified and expanded upon even into the 1980s [46–48], at the time, the mystery of the cause would have to wait for studies of uterine biochemistry to solve.

3.7 A Menstrual Toxin

Pliny the Elder (23–79 CE) warned that contact with menstrual fluid "turns new wine sour, crops touched by it become barren, grafts die, seed in gardens dry up, the fruit falls off tress, steel edges blunt and the gleam of ivory is dulled, bees die in their hives, even bronze and iron are at once seized by rust, and a horrible smell fills the air; to taste it drives dogs mad and infects their bites with an incurable poison" [49]. Menstruating women were so dangerous that some texts report that menstruating women were compelled to wear a bandage around the head during their flow to warn others of the danger. Despite this, menstrual blood was thought to be effective in the treatment of gout, sagging breasts, and other ailments (Fig. 3.19).

In modern times, these beliefs in toxicity were apparently proven by Béla Schick (most famous for the "Schick test" used to detect immunity to diphtheria toxin) when he documented a "menstrual toxin" that did, indeed, make flowers wilt [50, 51]. Subsequently Pickles, in 1957, reported that acetone and ether extracts of menstrual fluid contained a powerful "plain muscle stimulant" [52, 53]. These studies were expanded with the source of the stimulant localized to the sloughing endometrium [54–57]. By 1963, these agents had been identified as prostaglandins [58–60].

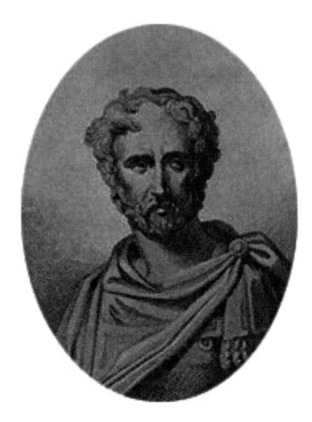

Fig. 3.19 Pliny the Elder,
Gaius Plinius Secundus
(23–August 25, 79 CE)

Fig. 3.20 The presence of a menstrual toxin was demonstrated when flowers that were not handled thrived, while the flowers that were handled by a menstruating woman wilted, as seen in Fig. 6, page 434 of Macht and Lubin [51]

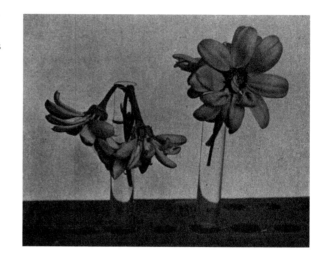

(This work would ultimately lead to the awarding of the 1982 Nobel Prize in Physiology or Medicine to Sune K. Bergström, Bengt I. Samuelsson, and John R. Vane (Fig. 3.20).)

The stage was now set for the connection between prostaglandins and uterine activity to be made. It came in 1965, when Pickles reported elevated levels of prostaglandin F_{2a} in the menstrual fluid of dysmenorrheic women [61]. The causative role of prostaglandin F_{2a} in dysmenorrhea was firmly established when studies duplicated dysmenorrhea-like pain and uterine activity after intravenous injection of prostaglandins [62]. The connection seemed complete between excess uterine prostaglandin F_{2a}, increased uterine activity, and the pain of dysmenorrhea. This understanding opened the possibility of interrupting the process at the source if the offending prostaglandins could be suppressed or counteracted.

3.8 Heavy Menstrual Flow

The relationship between painful and heavy menses has been acknowledged from antiquity to the modern era [63]. (Even the term menorrhagia is derived from Greek roots: *men*, month; *rhegyai*, to burst forth.) Because assessing the actual amount of blood lost during menstruation is problematic, recognition of abnormally heavy flow has often been difficult for the individual, and even more challenging to substantiate for others, including caregivers.

The Ebers Papyrus, written in the New Kingdom period (1550–1450 BCE), contains references thought to denote to the passage of blood clots during menstruation and prescribes "Nile earth from the water carrier, which you crush in honey and galena; put this on a dressing of fine linen and insert it into her vagina for four days." In the Hindu sacred books (the four Vedas of Brahma), written in about 1400 BCE, there is reference to heavy menstrual flow (*prodokoh*) (Fig. 3.21).

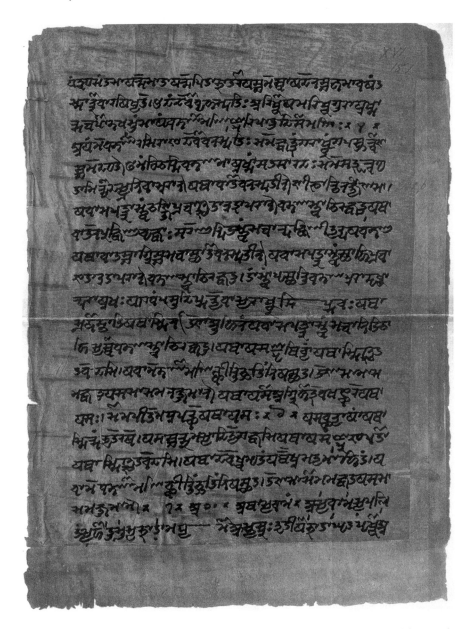

Fig. 3.21 The Vedas are ancient Sanskrit texts of Hinduism. Shown is a page from the *Atharvaveda*

In biblical times, the acknowledgment of menorrhagia is found in the story of the Haemorrhoissa as told in the Bible (Mark 5:24–34, Luke 8:42–48, and Matthew 9:19–22): A woman who had been suffering "hemorrhages" for 12 years approached Jesus and touched the hem of his cloak, thinking she would be made well. Jesus turned to the supplicant woman and said, "Daughter, your faith has made you well; go in peace, and be healed of your disease." (Fig. 3.22).

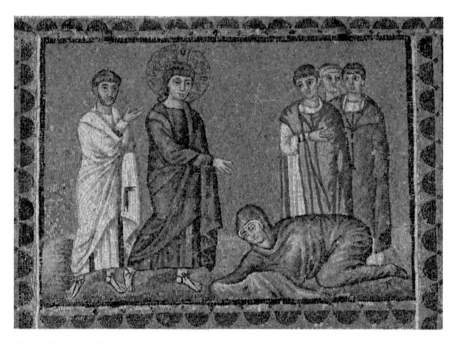

Fig. 3.22 Mosaic from the Basilica of Sant'Apollinare Nuovo, constructed in Ravenna, Italy in the early sixth century to be the palatine church of Theodoric, an Ostrogoth who conquered Italy, showing the story of the Haemorrhoissa

In the seventeenth century, it was commonly believed that physical exertion, such as dancing, would cause menstrual flow to be heavier. This lead to the recommendation that sanitary protections should be worn at occasions such as dances or balls, even if the woman was not currently menstruating [64]. By the nineteenth century, a more anatomic approach had displaced much, but not all, of the theories of causation. Thomas' textbook of gynecology lists fibrous tumors, cancer, polyps, and retained products of conception, in addition to "congestion" and "areolar hyperplasia" [65]. (The reference to the areola of the breast may be a carryover from the seventeenth-century idea that menstrual blood and breast milk were ultimately the same fluid [66], as evidenced by the absence of menses in breastfeeding women.)

During the seventeenth century, it was thought that the amount of blood lost during "normal" menses amounted to between one and two pints [67], in agreement with estimates attributed to Hippocrates. The actual establishment of the amount of blood lost during normal and abnormal menstruation did not occur until the work of Hallberg et al., in 1966 [68]. Their work showed that blood loss of more than 80 mL was associated (67% of the time) with anemia. This level then became the accepted upper limit of "normal" for menstrual bleeding. Unfortunately, studies have shown that there is a poor correlation between the blood loss measured in the research setting and the woman's perception of loss [69].

Key Points

- While it is probable that heavy, painful periods have been part of the lot of women throughout our history as a species, the views of society have influenced our perception of the process, cause, and treatments available.
- Many of the superstitions surrounding menstrual function eventually led to our understanding of uterine physiology. Examples include the role of prostaglandins (menstrual toxins) in uterine activity in creating menstrual pain and menorrhagia.
- With the recognition of the physiologic processes behind both normal and abnormal menstruation came not only the possibility of rational physiology-based therapies but also a change in the social perception of menstruation, allowing women to seek and receive appropriate treatment, without stigma.

References

1. Frandsen PJ. The menstrual "taboo" in ancient Egypt. J Near East Stud. 2007;66(2):81–106.
2. Read S. 'Thy righteousness is but a menstrual clout': sanitary practices and prejudice in early modern England. Early Modern Women. 2008;3:1–25. Available at: https://dspace.lboro.ac.uk/dspace-jspui/handle/2134/10271. Accessed 31 July 2017
3. Hampton J. The taboo of menstruation. Available at: https://aeon.co/essays/throughout-history-and-still-today-women-are-shamed-for-menstruating. Accessed 28 July 2017.
4. Whitelock A. Elizabeth's bedfellows: an intimate history of Elizabeth's court. London: Bloomsbury; 2014. p. 174.
5. Waller M. Sovereign ladies: the six reigning queens of England. New York: St. Martin's Press; 2006. p. 186.
6. Dickinson RL. Tampons as menstrual guard. JAMA. 1945;128(7):490–4.
7. Tizzano AP, Muffly TM. Historical milestones in female pelvic surgery, gynecology and female urology. In: Walters MD, Karram MM, editors. Urogynecology and reconstructive pelvic surgery. Philadelphia: Elsevier; 2015. p. 3–15.
8. Kudlien F. The seven cells of the uterus: the doctrine and its roots. Bull Hist Med. 1965;39(5):415–23.
9. Jacquart D, Thomasset C. Sexuality and medicine in the middle ages, Trans., Adamson M. Princeton: Princeton University Press; 1988. p. 34.
10. Power J. Essays on the female economy. London: Burgess and Hill; 1821.
11. Négrier C. Recherches anatomique et physiologiques sur les ovaires dans l'espèce humaine. Paris: Béchet, Jnr., et Labé; 1840.
12. Négrier C. Recueil des faits pour servir à l'histoire des ovaires et des affections hystériques de la femme. Angers; 1858.
13. Power J. An essay on the periodical discharge of the human female, with new views of its nature, causes, and influence on disease. To which are added directions for its management in the different stages of life. London: Burgess and Hill; 1832.
14. Jackson AR. A contribution to the relations of ovulation and menstruation. JAMA. 1884;3(14):365–72.
15. von Baer KE. De ovi mammalium et hominis genesi epistolam ad Academiam Imperialem Scientiarum Petropolitanam. Leipzig; 1827.
16. Mayer E. The intranasal treatment of dysmenorrhea. With a report of ninety-three cases. JAMA. 1914;62(1):6–8.
17. Origin and etymology of dysmenorrhea, Merriam-Webster on-line. Available at: https://www.merriam-webster.com/dictionary/dysmenorrhea. Accessed 19 May 2017.

18. McKay WJS. The history of ancient gynaecology. London: Balliere, Tindal and Cox; 1901.
19. Forbes RJ. Bitumen and petroleum in antiquity. Leiden (Holland): E. J. Brill; 1936. p. 92.
20. Symons P, Symons S. Bush heritage: an introduction to the history of plant and animal use by aboriginal people and colonists in the Brisbane and Sunshine Coast areas, Queensland, Australia. Nambour, Qld: Pat and Sim Symons; 1984. p. 106.
21. Coxe JR. The writings of Hippocrates and Galen, epitomised from the original Latin. Philadelphia: Lindsay and Blakiston; 1846.
22. Hippocates. Aphorisms, Section V. Adams F, trans. Available from: http://classics.mit.edu/Hippocrates/aphorisms.5.v.html. Accessed 23 May 2017.
23. Dioscorides. The Greek herbal of Dioscorides. Goodyer T, trans. Oxford, UK: Robert T. Gunther; 1933.
24. McKay WJS. The History of ancient gynæcology. London: Baillière, Tindall & Cox; 1901. p. 273.
25. Jenks EW. The practice of gynecology in ancient times. Trans Amer Gynec Soc. 1881;6:381.
26. Sultana A, ur Rahnam K. Effect of traditional dry cupping therapy on heavy menstrual bleeding in menorrhagia: a preliminary study. Int J Gen Trad Med. 2012;2(4):e33.
27. Ricci JV. One hundred years of gynecology 1800–1900. Philadelphia: Blakiston Co.; 1945. p. 522–4.
28. Emge LA. The problem of dysmenorrhea. Cal West Med. 1933;39:380–5.
29. Thomas TG. A practical treatise on the disease of women. Philadelphia: Henry C. Lea; 1872. p. 574.
30. Carstens JH. Some further observations on the use of the stem pessary for scanty menstruation, dysmenorrhea, infantile uterus and sterility. JAMA. 1904;43:1740–1.
31. Davenport FH. Uterine hæmorrhage: a consideration of some of the less common cause and their treatments. Boston Med Surg J. 1887;117(6):124–7.
32. Bell WB. Intrinsic dysmenorrhea. J Obstet Gynec Brit Emp. 1923;30(2):119–61.
33. Curtis AH. A text-book of gynecology. Philadelphia: WB Saunders; 1930., Fig. 164. p. 215.
34. Schatz F. Beiträge zur physiologischen geburtskunde. Arch Gynakol. 1872;3:58–144.
35. Schatz F. Beiträge zur physiologischen geburtskunde. Arch Gynak. 1872;4:34–111. 193–225, 418–456
36. Smith RP. A brief history of intrauterine pressure measurement. Acta Obstet Gynecol Scand. 1984;129(Suppl):1–24.
37. Rucker MP. Contractions of a non-pregnant multiparous human uterus. Am J Obstet Gynecol. 1925;9:255–7.
38. Novac E, Reynolds SRM. The cause of primary dysmenorrhea. JAMA. 1932;99:1466–72.
39. Krohn L, Lackener JE, Soskin S. The effect of the ovarian hormones on the human (nonpuerperal) uterus. Am J Obstet Gynecol. 1937;34:379–91.
40. Jacobson E, Lackner JE, Sinykin MB. Electrical and mechanical activity of the human non-pregnant uterus. Am J Obstet Gynecol. 1939;38:1008–20.
41. Jacobson E, Lackner JE, Sinykin MB. Activity of the human non-pregnant uterus. Am J Phys. 1940;53:407–17.
42. Wilson L, Kurzrok R. Studies on the motility of the human uterus in vivo. Endocrinology. 1938;23:79–86.
43. Wilson L, Kurzrok R. Uterine contractility in functional dysmenorrhea. Endocrinology. 1940;27:23–8.
44. Liessé A. L'Activité électrique de l'uterus dans la dysmenorrhee functionnelle. Gynec Obstet. 1948;47:850–1.
45. Woodbury RA, Torpin R, Child GP, et al. Myometrial physiology and its relation to pelvic pain. JAMA. 1947;134:1081–5.
46. Hendricks CH. Inherent motility patterns and response characteristics on the nonpregnant human uterus. Am J Obstet Gynecol. 1947;96:824–43.
47. Filler WW, Hall WC. Dysmenorrhea and its therapy: a uterine contractility study. Am J Obstet Gynecol. 1970;106:104–9.

48. Smith RP, Powell JR. The objective evaluation of dysmenorrhea therapy. Am J Obstet Gynecol. 1980;137:314–9.
49. Pliny: Natural History, vol 7,15:64. Available at: https://www.loebclassics.com/view/pliny_elder-natural_history/1938/pb_LCL352.549.xml. Accessed 23 May 2017.
50. Schick B. Menstrual toxins. Wein Klin Wschr. 1920;33:395–7.
51. Macht DI, Lubin DS. A phyto-pharmacological study of menstrual toxin. J Pharmacol Exp Ther. 1923;22(5):413–66.
52. Pickles VR. A plain muscle stimulant in the menstrual fluid. Nature (Lond). 1957;180:1198–9.
53. Pickles VR. Prostaglandins and dysmenorrhea: historical survey. Acta Obstet Gynecol Scand. 1979;87(Suppl):7–12.
54. Chambers PL, Pickles VR. Plain–muscle stimulants in extracts of menstrual fluid and of endometrial curettings. J Physiol. 1958;144:68–79.
55. Pickles VR. Some evidence that the endometrium produces a hormone that stimulates plain muscle. J Endocrinol. 1959;18:i–ii.
56. Pickles VR. Myometrial response to the menstrual plain-muscle stimulant. J Endocrinol. 1959;19:150–7.
57. Chambers PL. Further studies on the plain muscle stimulant present in human endometrium. J Endocrinol. 1960;20:vi–vii.
58. Clitheroe HJ, Pickles VR. The separation of the smooth-muscle stimulants in menstrual fluid. J Physiol. 1961;156:225–37.
59. Pickles VR, Hall WJ. Some physiological properties of the 'menstrual stimulant' substances A1 and A2. J Reprod Fertil. 1963;6:315–7.
60. Eglinton G, Raphael RA, Smith GN, Hall WJ, Pickles VR. The isolation and identification of two smooth muscle stimulants from menstrual fluid. Nature (Lond). 1963;200(960):993–5.
61. Pickles VR, Hall WJ, Best FA, Smith GN. Prostaglandins in endometrium and menstrual fluid from normal and dysmenorrheic subjects. J Obstet Gynaecol Br Comm. 1965;72:185–92.
62. Roth-Brandel U, Bygdman M, Wiqvist N. Effect of intravenous administration of prostaglandin E1 and F2a on the contractility of the non–pregnant women uterus in vivo. Acta Obstet Gynecol Scand. 1970;49(Supp 5):19–25.
63. M'Clintock AH. Clinical memoirs on diseases of women. Dublin: Fannin; 1863.
64. Freind J. Emmenologia, 1703, trans. Dale T, London: for T. Cox; 1729. p. 71.
65. Thomas TG. A practical treatise on the disease of women. Philadelphia: Henry C. Lea; 1872. p. 593.
66. Sadler I. The sicke womans private looking-glasse wherein methodically are handled all uterine affects, or diseases arising from the wombe; enabling women to informe the physician about the cause of their griefe. London: Printed by Anne Griffin, for Philemon Stephens, and Christopher Meridith, at the Golden Lion in S. Pauls Church-yard; 1636. p. 10.
67. Freind J. Emmenologia, 1703, trans. Dale T, London: for T. Cox; 1729. p. 1–4.
68. Hallberg L, Hogdahl AM, Nilsson L, Rybo G. Menstrual blood loss – a population study. Acta Obstet Gynaecol Scand. 1966;45:320–51.
69. Chimbira TH, Anderson ABM, Turnbull AC. Relation between measured menstrual loss and the patient's subjective assessment of loss, duration of bleeding, numbers of sanitary towels used, uterine weight and endometrial surface area. Br J Obstet Gynaecol. 1980;87:603–8.

Additional Resources

An interesting blog of menstrual topics: https://www.yahoo.com/style/great-moments-in-menstrual-history-c1262334095343670.html

The museum of menstruation has lots of history on menstruation, menstrual hygiene, and menstrual dysfunction: http://www.mum.org

An interesting doctoral dissertation on the history of menstrual hygiene in the United States: http://lib.dr.iastate.edu/cgi/viewcontent.cgi?article=11616&context=rtd

A good overview of the history of menstrual dysfunction: Rees MCP. Heavy, painful periods. In: Drife JO, editor. Dysfunctional uterine bleeding and menorrhagia. Clin Obstet Gynaecol. 1989;3(2):341–56.

A history of intrauterine pressure measurements can be found at: Smith RP. A brief history of intrauterine pressure measurement. Acta Obstet Gynecol Scand. 1984;129(Suppl):1–24.

Chapter 4
The Clinical Classification and Causes of Dysmenorrhea

4.1 Topic Overview

Unlike many conditions in medicine, the classification of painful menstruation into primary and secondary dysmenorrhea is not based on the temporal appearance of symptoms or the condition, as it is in primary and secondary amenorrhea, or primary and secondary infertility. The taxonomy of primary and secondary dysmenorrhea is based upon the absence or presence (respectively) of clinically identifiable causes. In both cases, a great deal is known about the pathophysiology underlying the development of menstrual pain. It is, therefore, not an issue of a lack of identifiable causation; it is the lack of *clinically* identifiable processes that drive the assignment.

As with most conditions in medicine, the best and most effective therapies are directed to the underlying pathologies. It was this foundational appreciation of pathophysiology that brought us to the ability to talk in terms of pain prevention, rather than pain relief for women with primary dysmenorrhea. The success achieved using this approach in dysmenorrhea can be viewed as the catalyst for similar successes in other areas of medicine ranging from interstitial cystitis to migraine headaches.

4.2 Classification Schemes

The recognized causes and the classifications of painful menstruation have evolved over many years. Nineteenth-century textbook authors such as Thomas [1], and many learned presentations of that era [2, 3], classified menstrual pain into neuralgic, congestive, inflammatory, obstructive, and membranous types, based upon the nature of the symptoms reported. In 1910, Bland suggested that the causes of dysmenorrhea could be looked upon as "general" and "local" [4]. Though a reasonable classification system, it still noted that, "among the general causes, environment and

© Springer International Publishing AG 2018
R.P. Smith, *Dysmenorrhea and Menorrhagia*,
https://doi.org/10.1007/978-3-319-71964-1_4

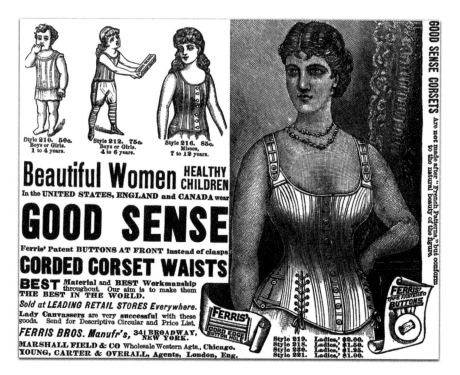

Fig. 4.1 An 1888 advertisement for corsets from Century Magazine; no. 6, 1888. Corsets of this type were still widely in use well into the twentieth century

hygiene play an important role. Women who live in cramped, unsanitary surroundings, with a scant supply of poor food and poor nutrition are likely to suffer from menstrual disorders." Bland went on to say, "Faulty wearing apparel with tight constrictions – corsets and bands around the waist – favors disturbance in the menstrual process" (Figs. 4.1 and 4.2).

By 1923, many textbooks had come to consolidate these ideas into "intrinsic" (an inherent abnormality of the structure or physiology of the uterus) or "extrinsic" (resulting from acquired pathologic processes) [5], though the classifications of "obstructive," "congestive," and "membranous" still could be found in the literature [6]. This move to uterine (intrinsic) and acquired (extrinsic) recognized that menstrual pain is broadly the result of multiple confluent causative pathways and not a unique entity unto itself. This was not to say the disability of menstrual pain was not a real entity, just that as a final common pathway, its presence was not diagnostic of the cause (Fig. 4.3).

Today's classification of dysmenorrhea into primary and secondary types came about as much from frustration as it did from insight. In secondary dysmenorrhea, the clinician, using their clinical diagnostic skills and little else, could identify a likely cause and direct therapies toward the problem. In the absence of such find-

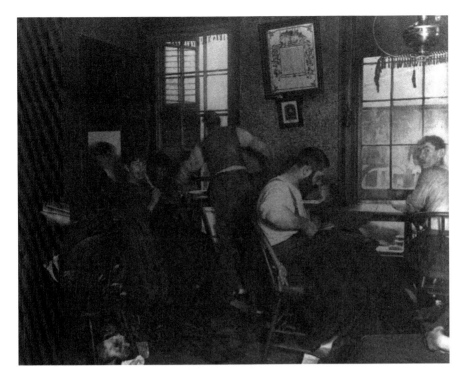

Fig. 4.2 Workers in a sweatshop in Ludlow Street Tenement, New York City c. 1889. Unfortunately, these conditions were common for young immigrant women of early reproductive age—those frequently affected by dysmenorrhea. (Image: Library of Congress, Prints and Photographs Division, Washington, DC.)

ings, therapy was often frustratingly ineffectual: Even the strongest opioids simply substituted one disability for another. This gave rise to great speculation about the process and the women who suffered. It was easier to explain the failures based upon the environment, temperament, or psyche than to profess an incomplete understanding. In short, that which is now called primary dysmenorrhea was simply "leftover" cases, often relegated to being psychogenic in origin and incurable in nature.

4.3 Secondary Dysmenorrhea

Pain is broadly classified into nociceptive (somatic and visceral) and non-nociceptive (neuropathic and sympathetic). In nociceptive pain, specific pain receptors are stimulated. These receptors sense temperature (hot/cold), mechanical stimuli (vibration, stretch, shear), and chemicals released from damaged cells though anoxia, inflammation, or chemical signaling molecules. The intensity of the pain

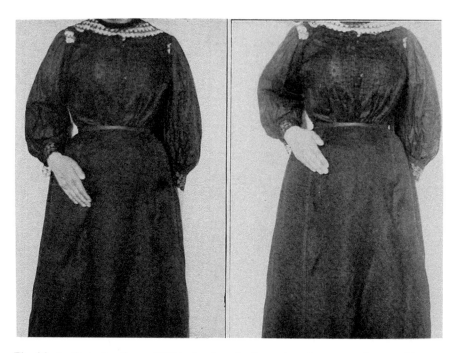

Fig. 4.3 An illustration from a 1907 textbook on the diagnosis and treatment of women illustrating the difference between the way pain in the adnexa (fallopian tubes or ovary) and the appendix would present. Knowledge such as this was often all the clinician had to go on when trying to find a cause for recurrent menstrual pain (Figs. 10 and 11 from Crossen [7])

Table 4.1 Nociceptive pain signaling

Type of receptor	Examples of painful stimuli
Thermal	Heat and cold
Mechanical	Excess pressure or mechanical deformation (e.g., crushing, tearing, stretching, shearing, etc.)
Chemical	Vasoactive amines, eicosanoids, inflammatory cytokines

perceived, indeed even the notice of the signal itself, is predicated upon a number of factors, the full extent of which are not fully understood. Variously referred to as a "pain threshold," factors such as fatigue, past experience, and expectations all play a role (Table 4.1).

Many pelvic pathologies can result in the generation of nociceptive neural signals. The most common mechanism for pelvic pathologies to cause pain is either stretch of peritoneal surfaces or through the liberation of inflammatory molecules. These pathologies may act in combination with normal physiologic changes to create discomfort, or they may act independently with their symptoms becoming more noticeable during menstruation.

Table 4.2 Causes of secondary dysmenorrhea

Intracavitary	Intramural	Extramural

Cervical stenosis and cervical lesions
Congenital abnormalities (outflow obstructions, uterine anomalies)
Endometrial polyps
Infection (chronic endometritis)
Intrauterine contraceptive devices (IUCDs)
Pedunculated leiomyomata
	Adenomyosis
	Tumors:
	  Leiomyomata,
	  sarcoma,
	  metastatic
		Endometriosis
		Inflammation and scarring (adhesions)
		Non-gynecologic causes:
		  Musculoskeletal, gastrointestinal, urinary
		"Pelvic congestive syndrome" (debated)
		Psychogenic (rare)
		Tumors:
		  Leiomyomas, benign, or malignant tumors of ovary, bowel, or bladder

Secondary dysmenorrhea is more common among women in the fourth and fifth decades of life, though occasionally occurring in adolescents, where endometriosis is more common. This predilection for the middle and later reproductive years parallels the prevalence of the typical dysmenorrhea pathologies across different ages. The possible etiologies of secondary dysmenorrhea may be broadly classified as being intrauterine and extrauterine, with intramural (within the uterine wall) bridging the two (Table 4.2).

Diffuse lower abdominal cramping, back or thigh pain, nausea, diarrhea, and headache may occur with either intrauterine or extrauterine sources of secondary dysmenorrhea. These symptoms are also common with primary dysmenorrhea, making their presence of little help in differentiating their origin. Extrauterine sources of secondary dysmenorrhea are the most likely to provide hints of their presence through additional, non-menstrual symptoms. Musculoskeletal, gastrointestinal, or urinary pathologies may cause symptoms at the time of menstruation, but their effects are rarely restricted to the time of flow. For example, irritable bowel syndrome often significantly worsens around the time of menstruation, but a careful history usually reveals postprandial cramping, food intolerance, or episodic diarrhea or constipation. Pelvic scarring (from surgery or inflammatory processes such as past infection) or endometriosis may cause overlooked symptoms of pain with intercourse, bowel movements, or physical activity. Intermenstrual spotting, often at midcycle, is sometimes found in patients with endometriosis. The process of somatization may focus symptoms on the pelvis that can worsen with the stress of menstruation, but it is rare for these patients not to exhibit symptoms at other times of the month or to not have signs suggesting stress, anxiety, depression, or personality disorders.

Intrauterine and intramural causes of dysmenorrhea tend to cause menstrual pain by disrupting the normal contractile activities of the uterus, the liberation of compounds such as prostaglandins, or both. Mechanical disruption of the muscle bundles of the uterine wall is thought to cause local spasms, ischemia, or abnormal stretch, all of which could result in the sensation of pain. This is most commonly associated with space-occupying processes, such as uterine leiomyomata, but may also be the mechanism behind some of the symptoms of adenomyosis (Fig. 4.4).

Fig. 4.4 With an incidence that increases with age, uterine leiomyomata are recognized source of both menstrual pain and heavy menstrual bleeding, even though the exact mechanism behind this disruption is not fully understood. The location of the fibroid, as shown in this 1913 illustration [8], plays a significant role in the character of the presenting symptoms, if any

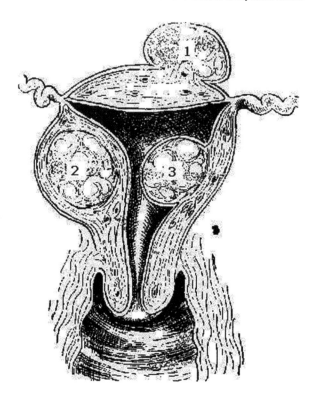

4.4   Primary Dysmenorrhea

As noted in the previous chapter, several lines of investigation have led us to understand that women with primary dysmenorrhea have abnormally high levels of prostaglandins (primarily prostaglandin $F_{2\alpha}$, $PGF_{2\alpha}$) [9] which stimulates abnormal levels and types of uterine contractile activity. Some studies have indicated a role for other molecules, such as vasopressin [10], but the role of these molecules appears limited.

Efforts to document the activity of the uterus predate even the perfection of the sphygmomanometer by Scipione Riva-Rocci, in 1896 [11]. Measurements of uterine activity in women with primary dysmenorrhea demonstrate rhythmic and dysrhythmic single and multiphasic contractions with peak pressures that can exceed 400 mmHg [12–14]. While there is no direct correlation between absolute pressure and pain [15], to place this in perspective, peak intrauterine pressures in labor are generally in the 70–100 mmHg range. Many women do report that the pain they experience with menses is more intense than that of their labors, a statement made more plausible by these pressure measurements (Figs. 4.5 and 4.6).

Studies have generally shown that the pain of primary dysmenorrhea is related to the work of the uterus and the quality of rest between contractions [12, 14, 15].

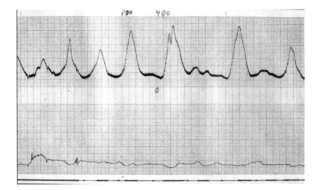

Fig. 4.5 Shown is a roughly 8 min recording of intrauterine (upper) and endocervical (lower) pressure during the early hours of a painful period. The pressure scale in the upper portion is from 0 to 400 mmHg. The baseline (resting pressure) varies between 60 and 80 mmHg, while the peak pressures approach 380 mmHg. The wide "blurred" portion of the tracing near baseline pressures represents the pulsatile inflow of blood, which is lost as intrauterine pressures exceed perfusion pressure. Carefully counting these small oscillations that make up the baseline portion of the tracing will reveal the patient's heart rate

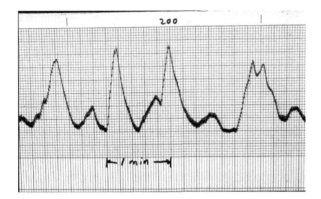

Fig. 4.6 In this tracing from a different patient, peak contraction pressures approximate 170 mmHg. The pulsatile inflow of blood may be more clearly seen here during the "rest" between contractions when pressures are 40–60 mmHg. Women who do not experience menstrual pain demonstrate resting pressures of 20–30 mmHg or less

Uterine work is reflected by parameters that include the number of contractions, their duration, magnitude, and the area under the pressure curve. Uterine rest includes the time between contractions and the baseline, or resting, pressure. This phase of reduced pressure is needed to allow for reperfusion of the uterus, providing re-oxygenation and the flushing of anaerobic waste. When uterine pressure exceeds arterial pressure, uterine ischemia develops and anaerobic metabolites accumulate, which stimulate type C pain neurons resulting in pain. Doppler studies show that women with primary dysmenorrhea have elevated uterine artery Doppler indices during menses, indicating higher resistance to blood flow in the uterine arteries, compared to women without dysmenorrhea [16, 17]. This matches what is seen in intrauterine pressure studies where the loss of pulsatile fluctuations in pressure indicative of arterial inflow is lost with increasing uterine pressure. These experimental findings match the intuitive idea that the more work the uterus performs, the more likely it is to generate both stretch and anoxic signals.

In addition to the mechanical processes that appear to induce the sensations of pain, there is data that suggests that $PGF_{2\alpha}$ itself can potentiate, if not originate, nociceptive pain signals [18–20]. This dual set of pathways to pain may explain the severity of discomfort experienced by these women.

4.5   Risk Factors

Few risk factors for the development of primary dysmenorrhea exist and most women with primary dysmenorrhea do not have predicting factors. Further, many of the risk factors that are proposed have been identified by association but lack supporting causal mechanism. They are also frequently general or unmodifiable in nature, such as age, making such recitations limited in their clinical utility.

In a systematic literature review that tried to identify risk factors for dysmenorrhea, age <30 years, body mass index <20 kg/m^2, smoking, menarche before age 12, longer menstrual cycles or duration of bleeding, irregular or heavy menstrual flow, and history of sexual assault were associated with higher rates of pain [21, 22]. While it has been proposed that there is some reduced risk with younger age at first childbirth and higher parity, this has not been consistently found and the relationship is weak. Regression analysis (when done) has suggested that age is a stronger factor in this change [23]. Increased levels of stress have demonstrated an increased risk and studies have reported that a family history of menstrual pain increases the risk by between 3.8- and 20.7-fold [24]. That said, studies have shown that other pain syndromes, such as migraine, also show familial tendencies [25].

Key Points
- The distinction between primary and secondary dysmenorrhea (based on clinically identified causation) is important for determining the most appropriate therapeutic plan.
- Through an understanding the pathophysiology of primary dysmenorrhea, safe, effective therapy is available which acts to alter the cause rather than treat the symptoms.
- The uterine activity seen in primary dysmenorrhea exceeds that seen in labor and results in intrauterine pressures well above tissue perfusion thresholds.
- The incidence of secondary dysmenorrhea parallels the underlying processes, such as the growth of uterine leiomyomata or endometriosis.
- Few risk factors have been identified for primary dysmenorrhea aside from age.

References

1. Thomas TG. A practical treatise on the disease of women. Philadelphia: Henry C. Lea; 1872. p. 574.
2. Levasseur F. Clinical observations on amenorrhea and dysmenorrhea. Milwaukee Med J. 1902;10(11):323–5.
3. Devasseur F. Clinical observations on amenorrhea and dysmenorrhea. J Med Sci. 1902;8:208–11.
4. Bland PB. Dysmenorrhea; its significance and treatment. J Med Soc NJ. 1910;6(12):591–4.
5. Bell WB. Intrinsic dysmenorrhea. J Obstet Gynec Brit Emp. 1923;30(2):119.
6. Caillé A. Postgraduate medicine, prevention and treatment of disease. New York and London: D. Appleton and Company; 1922. p. 661.
7. Crossen HS. The diagnosis and treatment of diseases of women. St. Louis: C.V. Mosby Medical Book and Pub. Co.; 1907. p. 8.
8. Gilliam T. A text-book of practical gynecology for practitioners and students. Philadelphia: FA Davis; 1913. p. 323.
9. Chan WY, Dawood MY, Fuchs F. Relief of dysmenorrhea with the prostaglandin synthetase inhibitor ibuprofen: effect on prostaglandin levels in menstrual fluid. Am J Obstet Gynecol. 1979;135:102–8.
10. Mechsner S, Grum B, Gericke C, Loddenkemper C, Dudenhausen JW, Ebert AD. Possible roles of oxytocin receptor and vasopressin-1α receptor in the pathomechanism of dysperistalsis and dysmenorrhea in patients with adenomyosis uteri. Fertil Steril. 2010;94(7):2541–6.
11. Smith RP. A brief history of intrauterine pressure measurement. Acta Obstet Gynecol Scand. 1984;129(Suppl):1–24.
12. Smith RP, Powell JR. The objective evaluation of dysmenorrhea therapy. Am J Obstet Gynecol. 1980;137:314–9.
13. Smith RP, Powell JR. Intrauterine pressure changes during Mefenamic acid treatment of primary spasmodic dysmenorrhea. Am J Obstet Gynecol. 1982;143:286–92.
14. Smith RP, Powell JR. Simultaneous objective and subjective evaluation of meclofenamate sodium in the treatment of primary dysmenorrhea. Am J Obstet Gynecol. 1987;157(3):611–6.
15. Smith RP, Heltzel J. Interrelation of analgesia and uterine activity in women with primary dysmenorrhea. A preliminary report. J Reprod Med. 1991;36:260–4.
16. Altunyurt S, Göl M, Altunyurt S, et al. Primary dysmenorrhea and uterine blood flow: a color Doppler study. J Reprod Med. 2005;50:251–5.
17. Dmitrović R. Transvaginal color Doppler study of uterine blood flow in primary dysmenorrhea. Acta Obstet Gynecol Scand. 2000;79:1112–6.
18. Gatta L, Piscitelli F, Giordano C, et al. Discovery of prostamide F2α and its role in inflammatory pain and dorsal horn nociceptive neuron hyperexcitability. PLoS One. 2012;7(2):e31111.
19. Grulović B, Pucelj MR, Krnić M, Kokić V. Impact of prostaglandin F2-alpha and tumor necrosis factor-alpha (TNF-alpha) on pain in patients undergoing thermal balloon endometrial ablation. Coll Antropol. 2013;37(4):1185–90.
20. Kunori S, Matsumura S, Mabuchi T, et al. Involvement of prostaglandin F 2 alpha receptor in ATP-induced mechanical allodynia. Neuroscience. 2009;163(1):362–71.
21. Latthe P, Mignini L, Gray R, et al. Factors predisposing women to chronic pelvic pain: systematic review. BMJ. 2006;332:749–55.
22. Hornsby PP, Wilcox AJ, Weinberg CR. Cigarette smoking and disturbance of menstrual function. Epidemiology. 1998;9:193–8.
23. Burnett MA, Antao V, Black A, et al. Prevalence of primary dysmenorrhea in Canada. J Obstet Gynaecol Can. 2005;27(8):765–70.

24. Ju H, Jones M, Mishra G. The prevalence and risk factors of dysmenorrhea. Epidemiol Rev. 2014;36:104–13.
25. Dzoljic E, Vlajinac H, Sipetic S, Marinkovic J, Grbatinic I, Kostic V. A survey of female students with migraine: what is the influence of family history and lifestyle? Int J Neurosci. 2014;124(2):82–7.

Additional Resources

More detailed coverage of many of the causes of secondary dysmenorrhea can be found here: Smith RP. Netter's obstetrics & gynecology. 3rd ed. Philadelphia: Elsevier; 2017.

Chapter 5
The Clinical Classification and Causes of Menorrhagia

5.1 Topic Overview

While harder to define, document, or diagnose, heavy menstrual bleeding still represents a significant cause of concern, imposition, and morbidity. As noted in Chap. 2, much of this occurs at a stage of life where its impact on education, productivity, or family relationships can have lifelong consequences. It is for this reason that The American College of Obstetricians and Gynecologists and others have recommended that menstruation be viewed as a "vital sign" [1].

Like menstrual pain, heavy menstrual bleeding is traditionally classified as primary or secondary based on the presence of clinically identifiable conditions known to be associated with menorrhagia. Heavy menstrual bleeding has recently been brought under a broader classification scheme that includes multiple forms of menstrual dysfunction—the PALM-COEIN system. There are many parallels between the older and newer classification systems, but the underlying key is the identification of causation wherever possible. Through that process, interventions will be much more effective at preventing or ameliorating the symptoms.

5.2 Classification Schemes

Because excessive menstrual flow can be dismissed as spurious or simply a part of a continuum of "normal flow" from light to heavy, separate classification schemes or investigations of causation have often lagged behind, or been lumped with, those of dysmenorrhea. Somewhat akin to the disease-centered teachings of older medical school curricula, heavy menstrual flow was frequently discussed as a possible outcome of specific pathologies, but not as a presenting complaint demanding a rich differential diagnosis [2]. This is like learning that the common cold and appendicitis can both cause fever but never fully considering what might be the causative

R.P. Smith, *Dysmenorrhea and Menorrhagia*,
https://doi.org/10.1007/978-3-319-71964-1_5

disease when confronted by a patient who is feverish. For the complaint of heavy menses, this unfortunately was a common issue. This left the clinician with few tools or constructs to use to identify possible pathology. To fill this void, there where even authors who advocated direct observation of the menstrual blood, both to verify the patient's report (as if they should not be trusted), but because it "further enables him to get certain clues from the inspection of the blood, which may certainly give much aid to the diagnosis. In addition to the amount of blood, there are the color [sic], the consistence, the formation of clots, and the mixture with other secretions and constituents of tissues to be considered" [3]. Note that the clinician was invariably identified as male, reflective of the gender distribution of the time (Fig. 5.1).

The causes proposed for the symptom of heavy menstrual bleeding have often been afterthoughts or driven by the prevailing medical fashion. For example, in the late nineteenth century, much was made of the role of inflammation in medicine, and thus, heavy menstrual flow got lumped in as a likely outcome of pelvic inflammation [5]. It could also be "the result of chronic congestion of the uterus, prolapses and other displacements, tumors, laceration of the neck of the uterus, disease of other organs and vegetations" [6]. (This latter list of causes was put forward by none other than John Harvey Kellogg, the inventor of Kellogg's Corn Flakes.) Even

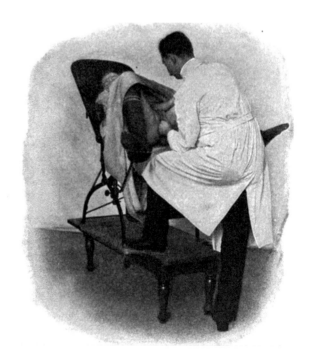

Fig. 5.1 The foundation of most classification schemes for heavy bleeding was, and remains, the findings on clinical examination of the patient [4]

"violent excitement, fright or a severe cold – may be responsible for the hemorrhage" [7]. Later authors have allocated the causes into organic, endocrinologic,
anatomic, and iatrogenic or have described them in terms of the role of the
hypothalamic-pituitary-ovarian axis (Fig. 5.2).

In part due to the common coexistence of menstrual pain and heavy flow, the
most common classification scheme for heavy menstrual bleeding became that of
primary and secondary, defined as with dysmenorrhea, based upon the presence or
absence of clinically identifiable pathology. This was the prevailing classification
scheme until 2011, when the International Federation of Gynecology and Obstetrics
(FIGO) introduced an overarching classification system for all menstrual disturbances, referred to by the acronym PALM-COEIN [8]. This classification system
provided a unification of older, poorly defined terms and classifies uterine bleeding
abnormalities by bleeding pattern as well as by etiology. The allocation of causes
into "structural" and "nonstructural" has many homologies to the older primary and
secondary classifications (Fig. 5.3).

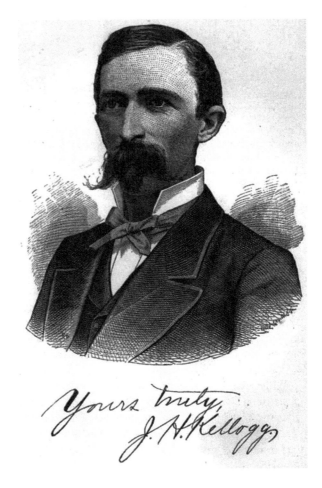

Fig. 5.2 None other than
John Harvey Kellogg, seen
here at roughly age 29,
weighed in on the causes
of heavy menstrual
bleeding

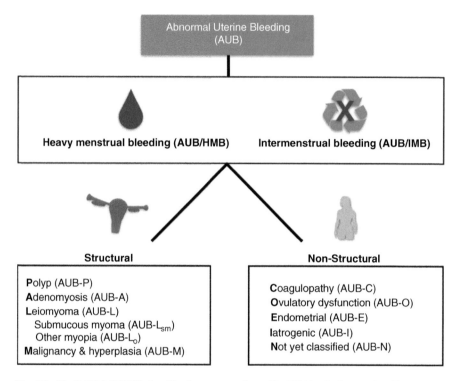

Fig. 5.3 The PALM-COEIN classification system adopted in 2011 by the International Federation of Gynecology and Obstetrics (FIGO) for abnormal uterine bleeding attempts to integrate both heavy and intermenstrual bleeding into a single common nomenclature and is based upon the character of the abnormal bleeding and structural versus nonstructural causes. Adapted from Munro et al. [8]

The FIGO system is extremely well suited to describing disturbances of menstrual cycle rhythm or duration. The system generally resolves the traditional allocation of cases without clinically obvious causation (primary menorrhagia) into "dysfunctional uterine bleeding" ascribed to "ovulatory dysfunction" (AUB/HMB-O) or "endometrial" (AUB/HMB-E). However, the more physiologic attribution of primary menorrhagia to an endometrial prostaglandin-mediated process that occurs most often in a setting of normal ovulatory function and normal endometrial histology makes the FIGO system problematic for discussions of heavy menstrual bleeding.

While the FIGO system has been endorsed by the American College of Obstetricians and Gynecologists as the preferred system [9], in the case of heavy rhythmic bleeding (our focus), the PALM-COEIN system offers little insight or nuance. For example, ovulatory disorders do not result in increased blood loss in the face of otherwise normal, regular menses, and they are generally excluded from the AUB/HMB label even though the pictorial depictions of PALM-COEIN would seem to include them. The system does not discriminate between endometrial hyperplasia and endometrial cancer, lumping them both under AUB-M. An accident of pregnancy, sometimes manifest as heavy vaginal bleeding, is neither periodic nor included in the FIGO classification, even though it presents as "intermenstrual bleeding." For this reason, the concept of primary versus secondary, identifiable versus cryptic causation, is still of value and will be used for the discussion below.

5.3 Secondary Menorrhagia

Traditionally, the causes of secondary menorrhagia have been those that were apparent to the skilled clinician through the use of the physical examination and a detailed history. Distortions of the uterus would portend the presence of uterine leiomyomata (AUB/HMB-L), a "woody" enlarged corpus suggested adenomyosis (AUB/HMB-A), a dilated cervix hinted at an intracavitary prolapsing myoma (AUB/HMB-L$_O$), and so forth. This resulted in lists of causes that were organized in the same manner as dysmenorrhea: intracavitary, intramural, and extramural. While conceptually useful, the majority of pathologies of greatest intrinsic threat to the patient are those within the uterine cavity. Studies suggest that among women with heavy menstrual bleeding, roughly 60% have intramural myomas, 30% have endometrial polyps, and 20% have extramural myomas [10]. A hysteroscopic study of women with heavy menstrual bleeding, stratified by measured blood loss, was reported by Fraser, in 1990, with similar ratios [11] (Table 5.1).

Intracavitary pathologies associated with heavy menstrual bleeding cause their symptoms through a disruption in the normal hemostatic regulatory systems of the intact endometrium. Abnormal spiral artery formation or function occurs in endometrial polyps and endometrial cancer, blunting the ability to control bleeding when

Table 5.1 Causes of secondary menorrhagia

Intracavitary	Intramural	Extramural
Arteriovenous malformations Endometrial hyperplasia Endometrial cancer Endometrial polyps Infection (chronic endometritis) Intrauterine contraceptive devices (IUCDs—Non-hormonal) Pedunculated leiomyomata Uterine sarcoma (rare)	Adenomyosis Tumors (leiomyomata, sarcoma, metastatic)	Blood dyscrasia (coagulopathy, e.g., von Willebrand disease, clotting factor deficiencies, immune thrombocytopenia, platelet function defects, and fibrinolytic pathway defects) Platelet dysfunction (uremia, cirrhosis, myeloma, polycythemia, thrombocytopenia) Spurious (inaccurate perception, fallacious)

the surface becomes unstable and is lost. Uterine arteriovenous malformations are a rare cause of heavy menstrual bleeding [12, 13] and should be suspected when an invasive procedure seems to aggravate the problem. Patients with these malformations typically have a history of failed intrauterine pregnancies, uterine curettage, cesarean delivery, or cesarean scar pregnancies.

Pressure from the narrow base of polyps, or mechanical disruption from a leiomyomata's growth, may result in venous stasis. The increased endometrial surface area overlying a mural leiomyoma, or the increased vascularity associated with its growth, can contribute to heavier menstrual bleeding. The thickened endometrium of endometrial hyperplasia provides abundant amounts of arachidonic acid when sloughed endometrial cell walls are metabolized by phospholipase. Cellular irritation caused by a non-hormonal intrauterine contraceptive device or endometritis promotes the formation or liberation of inflammatory cytokines and prostaglandins. In each case, the pathway that leads to heavy menstrual bleeding is reasonably well understood or can be plausibly hypothesized, even if the factors that lead to the underlying pathology are not (Fig. 5.4).

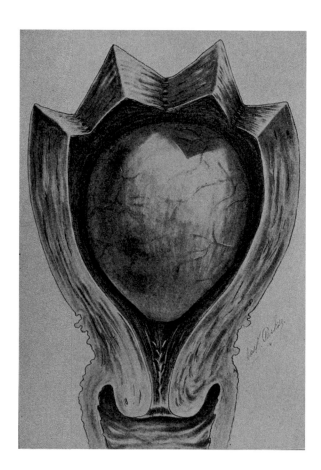

Fig. 5.4 An example of a large intracavitary leiomyoma attached to the posterior uterine wall and distorting the uterus as seen in a 1905 illustration [14]

5.4   Primary Menorrhagia

Unlike primary dysmenorrhea where a disturbance in prostaglandin production is essentially the only cause of pain that does not have a specific clinical finding, in primary menorrhagia a number of cryptic (not clinically obvious) causes must be considered in the absence of clinical findings. For example, excessive menstrual bleeding can be the result of a coagulopathy (AUB/HMB-C) or iatrogenic anticoagulation (AUB/HMB-I), lack outward signs, but these cases are rarely without other symptoms, a suggestive history, or associated findings. Heavy menstrual flow can be the result of endometrial changes that are not apparent on physical examination, though it could be argued that they may be documented by ultrasonography in many cases. In the case of new onset of heavy bleeding in older patients, the possibility of endometrial cancer (AUB/HMB-M) must always be considered even in the absence of palpable uterine changes. Given the availability and ease with which both endometrial histologic sampling and ultrasonographic imaging are available, many argue that these modalities should be included with the physical examination in classifying menorrhagia into primary and secondary types. For this discussion, we will follow that convention as well.

Although menorrhagia may be due to systemic or pelvic disease, no pathology is found in 50% of cases, and the majority of women with menorrhagia have normal ovulatory cycles [15, 16]. The recognized cause for heavy menstrual bleeding in these women is elevated levels of thromboxane A_2 (TXA_2) and prostaglandin E_2 (PGE_2). Studies show that women with menorrhagia have elevated total levels of prostaglandins (PGE_2, $PGF_{2\alpha}$, and PGI_2) and an increased ratio of PGE_2 to $PGF_{2\alpha}$ [17–19]. The role of leukotrienes has been studied in menorrhagia, but no correlation was found between leukotriene release in either the endometrium or myometrium and menstrual blood loss [20].

For most patients, the excess production of TXA_2 and $PGF_{2\alpha}$ is driven by the availability of the arachidonic acid substrate used by cyclooxygenase, lipoxygenase, and epoxygenases. Any process, including the secretory changes associated with normal ovulatory cycles, that results in a lush endometrium, will provide larger amounts of that substrate.

5.5   Risk Factors

In the literature, established risk factors for menorrhagia include increased age [21], premenopausal leiomyomata [22], and endometrial polyps [23]. Because bleeding is the most common presenting symptom for these pathologies, it must be recognized that calling them risk factors is of little clinical utility. Parity, body mass index, exercise, education level, and smoking have not been established as risk factors [21, 24], though weight has been associated with longer cycle length [25]. In some studies, up to 20% of women with heavy menstrual bleeding will be found to have an underlying inherited bleeding disorder [26–28]. A history of sexual assault is twice as common among women with symptoms of dysmenorrhea, heavy menses, and sexual dysfunction as compared with women without such complaints [29], and this possibility should be explored with the patient.

Women with heavy menstrual bleeding have been reported to have increased expression of cyclooxygenases (COX-1, COX-2) and increased endometrial responsiveness to stimulation by prostaglandins [30]. This observation would suggest a heritable propensity to heavy menstrual bleeding, though none has been conclusively demonstrated.

Key Points
- The historic classification of the causes of heavy menstrual bleeding parallels that of dysmenorrhea: primary and secondary.
- The PALM-COEIN classification of abnormal menstrual bleeding is useful for most forms of abnormal bleeding patterns but is less useful for defining the causes of heavy, but rhythmic, menstrual bleeding.
- Unlike primary dysmenorrhea, when the cause of heavy menstrual bleeding is not immediately clinically apparent, further evaluations of the endometrium and uterine cavity should be performed before presuming the absence of significant pathology.
- The only reliable risk factors for heavy menstrual flow are those associated with the causative pathologies of secondary menorrhagia.

References

1. American College of Obstetricians and Gynecologists. Menstruation in girls and adolescents: using the menstrual cycle as a vital sign. Committee Opinion No. 651. Obstet Gynecol. 2015;126:e143–6.
2. Champneys FH. Some points in the natural history of uterine fibroids. Lancet. 1900:147–50.
3. Edge F. Diagnosis of bleeding from the female genitals. Birmingham Med Rev. 1898;44:355–65.
4. Winter G, Ruge C, Clark JG. Text-book of gynecological diagnosis. Philadelphia & London: JB Lippincott Co.; 1909. front plate
5. Montgomery EE. Endometritis; subinvolution; retroversion; dilation, curetting and vaginal fixation. Ther Gazette. 1895;19(2):73–7.
6. Kellogg JH. Menorrhagia – uterine hemorrhage. In: The home book of modern medicine: a family guide in health and disease, vol. 2. Battle Creek, MI: The Good Health Publishing Company; 1909. p. 1332–4.
7. Winter G, Ruge C, Clark JG. Text-book of gynecological diagnosis. Philadelphia & London: JB Lippincott Co.; 1909. p. 604–14.
8. Munro MG, Critchley HO, Broder MS, Fraser IS. FIGO classification system (PALM-COEIN) for causes of abnormal uterine bleeding in nongravid women of reproductive age. FIGO Working Group on Menstrual Disorders. Int J Gynaecol Obstet. 2011;113:3–13.
9. American College of Obstetricians and Gynecologists. Diagnosis of abnormal uterine bleeding in reproductive-aged women. Practice Bulletin No. 128. Obstet Gynecol. 2012;120:197–206.
10. Clevenger-Hoeft M, Syrop CH, Stovall DW, et al. Sonohysterography in premenopausal women with and without abnormal bleeding. Obstet Gynecol. 1999;94(4):516–20.

11. Fraser IS. Hysteroscopy and laparoscopy in women with menorrhagia. Am J Obstet Gynecol. 1990;162(5):1264–9.
12. Hoffman MK, Meilstrup JW, Shackelford DP, Kaminski PF. Arteriovenous malformations of the uterus: an uncommon cause of vaginal bleeding. Obstet Gynecol Surv. 1997;52:736–40.
13. Nicholson AA, Turnbull LW, Coady AM, Guthrie K. Diagnosis and management of uterine arterio-venous malformations. Clin Radiol. 1999;54:265–9.
14. Findley P. The diagnosis of diseases of women. 2nd ed. Philadelphia and New York: Lea Brothers & Co.; 1905. p. 313. Fig. 134
15. Haynes PJ, Anderson ABM, Turnbull AC. Patterns of menstrual blood loss in menorrhagia. Res Clin Forums. 1979;1:73–8.
16. Chimbira TH, Anderson AB, Turnbull A. Relation between measured menstrual blood loss and patient's subjective assessment of loss, duration of bleeding, number of sanitary towels used, uterine weight and endometrial surface area. Br J Obstet Gynaecol. 1908;87(7):603–9.
17. Willman EA, Collins WP, Clayton SG. Studies in the involvement of prostaglandins in uterine symptomatology and pathology. Br J Obstet Gynaecol. 1976;83:337–41.
18. Smith SK, Abel MH, Kelly RW, Baird DT. Prostaglandin synthesis in the endometrium of women with ovular dysfunctional uterine bleeding. Br J Obstet Gynaecol. 1981;88:434–42.
19. Cameron IT, Leask R, Kelly RW, Baird DT. Endometrial prostaglandins in women with abnormal menstrual bleeding. Prostaglandins Leukot Med. 1987;29:24957.
20. Rees MCP, Di Marzo V, Tippins JR, Morris HP, Turnbull AC. Leukotriene release by endometrium and myometrium throughout the menstrual cycle in dysmenorrhoea and menorrhagia. J Endocrinol. 1987;113:291–5.
21. Janssen CA, Scholten PC, Heintz AP. Menorrhagia—a search for epidemiological risk markers. Maturitas. 1997;28:19–25.
22. Wegienka G, Baird DD, Hertz-Picciotto I, et al. Self-reported heavy bleeding associated with uterine leiomyomata. Obstet Gynecol. 2003;101:431–7.
23. DeWaay DJ, Syrop CH, Nygaard IE, Davis WA, Van Voorhis BJ. Natural history of uterine polyps and leiomyomata. Obstet Gynecol. 2002;100:3–7.
24. Gordley LB, Lemasters G, Simpson SR, et al. Menstrual disorder and occupational, stress, and racial factors among military personnel. J Occup Environ Med. 2000;42(9):871–81.
25. Hartz AJ, Barboriak PN, Wong A, et al. The association of obesity with infertility and related menstrual abnormalities in women. Int J Obes. 1979;3(1):57–73.
26. Shankar M, Lee CA, Sabin CA, Economides DL, Kadir RA. Von Willebrand disease in women with menorrhagia: a systematic review. BJOG. 2004;111:734–40.
27. American College of Obstetricians and Gynecologists. Von Willebrand disease in women. Committee Opinion No. 580. Obstet Gynecol. 2013;122:1368–73.
28. Davies J, Kadir RA. Heavy menstrual bleeding: an update on management. Thromb Res. 2017;151(Suppl 1):S70–7.
29. Golding JM, Wilsnack SC, Learman LA. Prevalence of sexual assault history among women with common gynecologic symptoms. Am J Obstet Gynecol. 1998;179(4):1013–9.
30. Smith OP, Jabbour HN, Critchley HO. Cyclooxygenase enzyme expression and E series prostaglandin receptor signaling are enhanced in heavy menstruation. Hum Reprod. 2007;22:1450–6.

Additional Resources

A good overview of the diagnosis and management of abnormal bleeding can be found at:
American College of Obstetricians and Gynecologists. Diagnosis of abnormal uterine bleeding in reproductive-aged women. Practice Bulletin No. 128. Obstet Gynecol. 2012;120:197–206.

Chapter 6
The Role of Prostaglandins in Dysmenorrhea and Menorrhagia

6.1 Topic Overview

First identified in prostatic secretions, the 20-carbon eicosanoids that make up the prostaglandins, prostacyclins, and thromboxanes, perform critical cellular and regulatory functions throughout the body. These molecules are produced from arachidonic acid by the enzymatic action of cyclooxygenase and other enzymes. Part of the broader class of paracoids and autacoids, biological agents that function as local hormones, have a short half-life, and act very near the point of synthesis; these molecules play important roles in both physiology and pathology. Prostaglandins mediate inflammatory and anaphylactic reactions, the prostacyclins are active in clotting and the resolution phase of inflammation, and the thromboxanes are mediators of vasoconstriction. In the uterus, prostaglandins are critical to vascular tone, normal blood clotting, and orchestrating labor and parturition.

Because of the role that excess prostaglandins play in both dysmenorrhea and heavy menstrual bleeding, an understanding of their creation, action, and involvement in reproduction is foundational. The effective treatments of dysmenorrhea and menorrhagia used today are based upon interdicting the biochemical cascades described here.

6.2 The Formation and Action of Prostaglandins

Prostaglandins, prostacyclins, and thromboxanes are all members of a subclass of eicosanoids referred to as prostanoids. Prostanoids are derivatives of arachidonic acid, a polyunsaturated omega-6 fatty acid. Specific prostanoids are named with a letter indicating the type of ring structure, followed by a number indicating the number of double bonds in the hydrocarbon "tail" structure. A Greek

© Springer International Publishing AG 2018
R.P. Smith, *Dysmenorrhea and Menorrhagia*,
https://doi.org/10.1007/978-3-319-71964-1_6

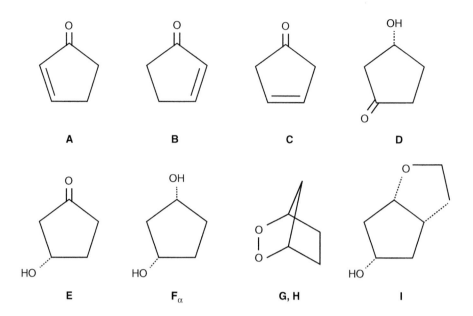

Fig. 6.1 By convention, the naming of prostaglandins is based upon the functional groups of the cyclopentane ring, while the number reflects number of double bonds in the trailing carbon chains. The type formed is dependent on the character of the fatty acid substrate and the enzymatic pathway followed

subscript (α or β) is used with prostaglandins of the PGF series to describe the stereochemistry of the hydroxyl group on carbon 9 (Fig. 6.1).

Arachidonic acid is classified as a carboxylic acid, with a 20-carbon chain and four *cis*-double bonds; the first double bond is located at the sixth carbon from the omega (COOH) end. Arachidonic acid is found in cell walls throughout the body, with skeletal muscle containing an especially large amount, accounting for roughly 10–20% of the phospholipid fatty acid content. Most of the arachidonic acid in humans originates from dietary animal sources (meat, eggs, or dairy), though it can also be synthesized from linoleic acid. Arachidonic acid acts as the feedstock for a number of biochemical reactions. For the purposes of this discussion, we will focus on the pathways referred to as the arachidonic acid cascade—those characterized by the enzymatic actions of epoxygenases, lipoxygenases, and cyclooxygenase—with the bulk of our focus on the latter (Fig. 6.2).

Arachidonic acid can be metabolized by lipoxygenases (primarily arachidonate 5-lipoxygenase) into several leukotrienes (hydroperoxides), which are important mediators of immune responses. Leukotrienes, especially leukotriene D_4 (LTD$_4$), trigger contractions in the smooth muscles lining the bronchioles, and it is their overproduction that is a major cause of inflammation in asthma [2]. In inflammation, the production of leukotrienes is usually accompanied by the formation of histamine, which also acts as an inflammatory mediator. Leukotrienes

Fig. 6.2 Arachidonic acid is liberated from the cell wall by the action of phospholipase (primarily A$_2$ but with C as well), released from the lysosome. This release is suppressed by increased levels of progesterone. Cortisol inhibits the actions of phospholipase and stabilizes the cell membrane [1]

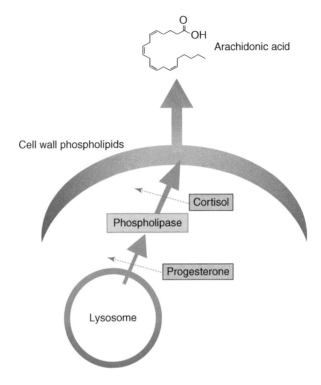

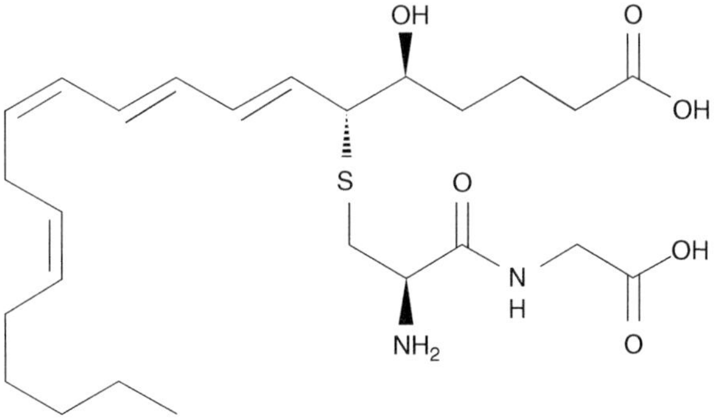

Fig. 6.3 Leukotriene D$_4$ is a cysteinyl leukotriene and is the major regulator of the smooth muscles lining the bronchioles. Overproduction is a major factor in the symptoms of asthma and allergic rhinitis

Leukotriene D$_4$

may also be produced from the essential fatty acid eicosapentaenoic acid (EPA) by the same metabolic pathway used to metabolize arachidonic acid, producing leukotriene B$_5$ (Fig. 6.3).

Leukotrienes are notable for the common inclusion of the amino acid cysteine in their structure, specifically LTC$_4$, LTD$_4$, LTE$_4$, and LTF$_4$. These cysteinyl leukotrienes make up the slow-reacting substance of anaphylaxis. The lipoxygenase

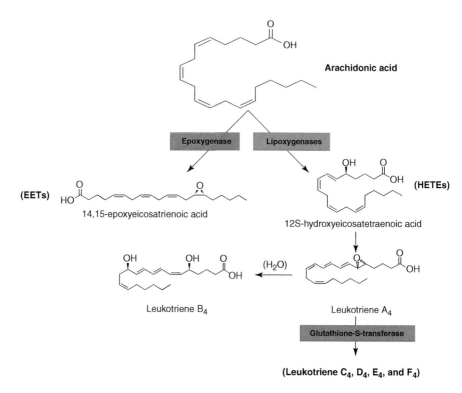

Fig. 6.4 Arachidonic acid can be metabolized by what is referred to as the second and third pathway of eicosanoid production (right to left above). These produce the leukotrienes, hydroxyeicosatetraenoic acids (HETEs) and epoxyeicosatrienoic acids (EETs)

pathway is most active in leukocytes and other immunocompetent cells, including mast cells, eosinophils, neutrophils, monocytes, and basophils (Fig. 6.4).

Epoxygenases (a large family of membrane-bound heme-containing cytochrome P450 enzymes) metabolize arachidonic acid into epoxyeicosatrienoic acids (EETs) that are also short-lived cellular signaling molecules. This represents the "third pathway" of eicosanoid metabolism. The cytochrome epoxygenases generally act on a wider range of polyunsaturated fatty acids than just arachidonic acid, forming a broader range of metabolites than are formed in the first and second pathways of eicosanoid production. Epoxyeicosatrienoic acids prevent arterial occlusive diseases such as heart attacks and thrombotic strokes. This occurs through their antihypertension action and anti-inflammatory effects on blood vessels, their inhibition of platelet activation, and their promotion of pro-fibrinolytic removal of thrombi [3]. Studies have implicated the EETs in the pathological growth of certain types of cancer and in the physiological, and possibly pathological, perception of neuropathic pain [4, 5]. This "peripheral sensitization" potentiates the pain-producing activity of bradykinin and other autacoids [6] (Fig. 6.5).

Fig. 6.5 Chronic, debilitating neuropathic pain may be mediated by epoxyeicosatrienoic acids. An 1896 image of pain from a home health textbook by Foote [7]

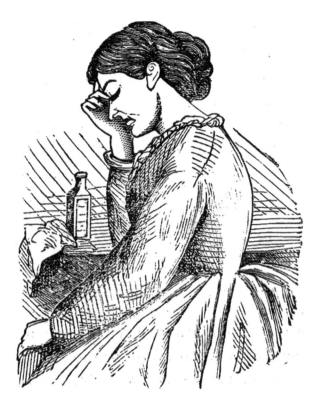

Within the uterus, the most important eicosanoid production pathway is that of the prostanoids. Cyclooxygenase (COX), officially known as prostaglandin-endoperoxide synthase (PTGS), is the pivotal enzyme in this process. This enzyme inserts two atoms of oxygen into arachidonate to yield a 15-hydroperoxy-9,11-endoperoxide with a substituted cyclopentane ring (prostaglandin G_2, PGG_2). This is reduced to its 15-hydroxy analog, prostaglandin H_2 (PGH_2). While both PGG_2 and PGH_2 have intrinsic biologic activity as vasodilators and aggregators of platelets, they are inherently unstable and are quickly metabolized into the more important prostanoids: the thromboxanes, prostacyclin, and the prostaglandins (Fig. 6.6).

Cyclooxygenase exists in two primary forms: COX-1, which is always present in tissues, and COX-2 which is induced by physiologic stimuli such as cytokines, tumor promoters, tissue damage, and growth factors. A third form, COX-3, has been described but plays a much less biologically important role. The two main isoenzymes have approximately 60% sequence homology and nearly identical catalytic sites. They are similar in structure, differing in that COX-2 has a larger molecular pocket near the active site due to an isoleucine to valine substitution. The result is that COX-2 can be more permissive in utilizing fatty acids other than arachidonic acid. This difference also allows for the possibility of selective blockade of the

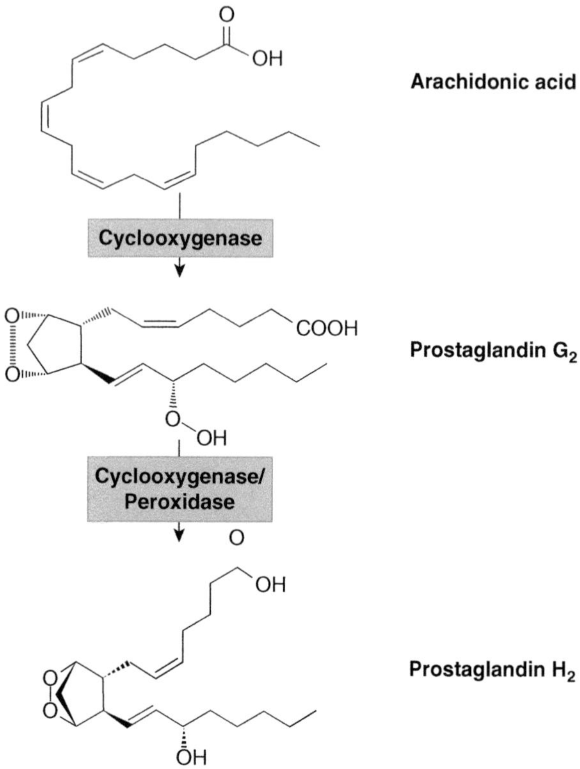

Fig. 6.6 Prostaglandins G_2 and H_2 are produced from arachidonic acid. The reaction, an oxygenation, requires the enzyme cyclooxygenase (COX-1 or COX-2), which inserts two molecules of O_2 into the C-H bonds of the arachidonic acid to form PGG_2, which is quickly converted to PGH_2 by shedding a single oxygen. (Note: The enzymes most critical to uterine function and dysfunction will be consistently shown in light blue, as shown here)

Arachidonic acid

Cyclooxygenase

Prostaglandin G_2

Cyclooxygenase/ Peroxidase

Prostaglandin H_2

active site using molecules of different sizes, as seen in selective COX-1 and COX-2 inhibitors. Both enzymes catalyze the same reaction, adding two molecules of oxygen to arachidonic acid (Fig. 6.7).

In general, COX-1 is used for "housekeeping" (homeostatic) purposes, responding quickly to circulating hormones, which require constant monitoring and regulation. In contrast, COX-2 is an inducible enzyme that is not normally present in tissues other than the kidney and brain. It is expressed under a wide range of extracellular and intracellular stimuli, such as cytokines, tissue shear stress, growth factors, and tumor promoters. Cyclooxygenase-2 is able to utilize much lower concentrations of arachidonic acid and substrates other than the free acid. Both COX-1 and COX-2 reside in the endoplasmic reticular membrane, but not in the cellular plasma or mitochondrial membranes (Table 6.1).

The three classes of prostanoids formed by cyclooxygenase action have distinctive rings in the center of the molecule. The compounds derived from PGH (as PGH_1, PGH_2, or PGH_3) have a 5-carbon ring, bridged by two oxygens (a peroxide). The subsequent prostaglandins contain a single, unsaturated 5-carbon ring. In prostacyclins, this ring is conjoined to another oxygen-containing ring, while in thromboxanes the ring becomes a 6-member ring with one oxygen (Fig. 6.8).

Fig. 6.7 Crystal structure of arachidonic acid bound in the cyclooxygenase active site of cyclooxygenase-1. (Molecular graphics images produced using the UCSF Chimera package from the Resource for Biocomputing, Visualization, and Informatics at the University of California, San Francisco)

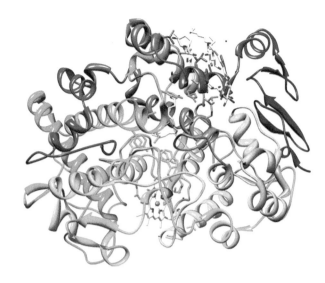

Table 6.1 Factors that affect prostaglandin synthesis[a]

Stimulatory	Inhibitory
Ca^{++}	Lipocortin
Platelet-activating factor	Endogenous inhibitor of PG synthesis (EIPS)
ß-agonists	Chorion phospholipase A_2 inhibitor
Estrogen	(lipocortin VI)
Cortisol	Cortisol
Epidermal growth factor	Progesterone
Transforming growth factor a	Estrogen
Interleukin-1 α and ß	Interferon α
Lipopolysaccharide	
Tumor necrosis factor (TNF)	
Adrenocorticotropin	
Corticotropin-releasing factor	
Placental PGDH inhibitor	

[a]It should be noted that some agents (e.g., estrogen, cortisol) may be either stimulatory or inhibitory depending on the tissue and other factors

Prostacyclin (PGI_2) and the thromboxanes are synthesized directly from PGH_2 by prostacyclin synthase and thromboxane-A synthase, respectively. Prostacyclin is the main prostanoid formed in endothelial and smooth muscle cells, while thromboxane-A is the predominate product in platelets and lung tissue. Activated platelets synthesize TXA_2 almost exclusively through the actions of COX-1. Increased amounts of TXA_2 amplify further platelet activation and recruitment. It is the irreversible inhibition of COX-1 by aspirin that is the mechanism behind aspirin's cardioprotective effects. Prostacyclin is the major platelet inhibitory prostanoid. It is synthesized by COX-2, and to a lesser degree by COX-1, in vascular endothelial and

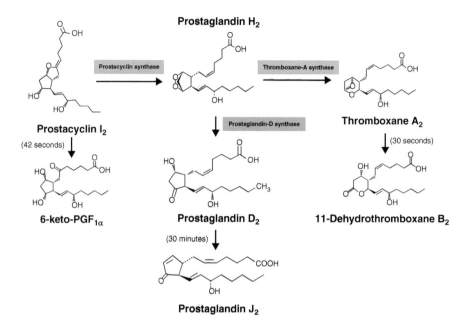

Fig. 6.8 Prostaglandin H_2 is converted to prostacyclin I_2 and thromboxane A_2 through the action of the enzymes shown. These two compounds are particularly important in the regulation of bleeding in other parts of the body, but menstrual bleeding relies on other mechanisms for control. (See Chap. 1.) Both have half-lives that are measured in seconds

smooth muscle cells. In most tissues, it is the balance between PGI_2 and TXA_2 that modulates platelet adhesion and clotting.

Prostaglandin E_2, also known as dinoprostone, is the most common and most biologically potent of mammalian prostaglandins. It is also, perhaps, the best studied of all of the prostaglandins. It is produced from PGH_2 by prostaglandin E synthase, which has at least three forms that are structurally and biologically distinct. It appears that microsomal prostaglandin E synthase-1 (MPES-1) is the key enzyme in the formation of PGE_2. From mediating inflammation and inducing fever, to increasing vascular permeability and stimulating bone resorption, PGE_2 carries out regulatory functions throughout the body. It is a key mediator of inflammation and pain in both rheumatoid and osteoarthritis. It is a direct vasodilator, relaxing vascular smooth muscle, and it inhibits the release of noradrenaline from sympathetic nerve terminals. Like the EETs, PGE_2 appears to be capable of causing hyperalgesia [8]. Formed in the interior of cells, PGE_2 exits the cell through both diffusion and active membrane transport mechanisms [9]. The biologic half-life of PGE_2 is 8.8 (±3.4) h, though under some conditions this may be as short as 2 h [10] (Fig. 6.9).

Prostaglandin $F_{2\alpha}$ may be formed directly from PGH_2 by endoperoxide F reductase, but most often it is made from PGE_2 by PGE 9-ketoreductase. Prostaglandin $F_{2\alpha}$ is a potent smooth muscle stimulant in the vascular wall, the gut, and the myometrium. Along with oxytocin, it is critical to the progress of labor. Prostaglandin $PGF_{2\alpha}$ also has an important pro-inflammatory function, especially in chronic inflammatory diseases such as rheumatoid arthritis. The half-life of $PGF_{2\alpha}$ is 15.0

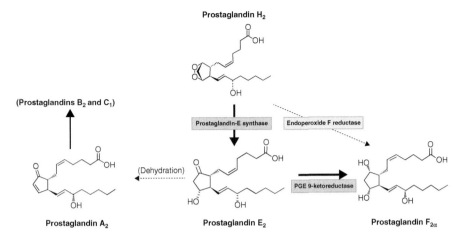

Fig. 6.9 The primary prostaglandins made in the endometrium and myometrium are PGE_2 and $PGF_{2\alpha}$

Table 6.2 General function of prostaglandins

Type	General function
PGl_2	Vasodilation Inhibition of platelet aggregation Bronchodilation
PGE	(Hyperalgesia and fever)
PGE_1	Bronchoconstriction Gastrointestinal tract smooth muscle contraction
PGE_2	Bronchodilation Gastrointestinal tract smooth muscle relaxation Vasodilation
PGE_3	Decreased gastric acid secretion Increased gastric mucus production Uterine contraction in pregnancy Gastrointestinal tract smooth muscle contraction
$PGF_{2\alpha}$	Uterine contraction Bronchoconstriction

(± 8.2) h, though when exposed to decidual cells, this may be as short as 2 h [10] and on the order of 1 min in blood plasma.

Prostaglandin A_2 activates intrinsic apoptotic pathways by directly stimulating mitochondrial outer membrane permeabilization to release cytochrome C, and exhibits potent cellular antiproliferative activity in vivo and in vitro. It inhibits cell growth by blocking cell cycle at the G1 and G2/M phase by inhibiting G1 phase cyclin-dependent kinases [11] downregulating cyclin D1 [12].

All eicosanoids function locally at the site of synthesis, through receptor-mediated G-protein-linked signaling pathways. Eicosanoids, including the prostanoids, are not stored within cells but are synthesized as required in response to hormonal or other stimuli. The biologic effects of the eicosanoids are a function of their isoform and the receptors found on the cell membrane of the tissue under consideration (Table 6.2).

6.3 Prostaglandins in Reproduction, Dysmenorrhea, and Heavy Menstrual Bleeding

In the uterus, it is the cyclooxygenase pathway of arachidonic acid metabolism that is most active. In the endometrium, PGE_2 and $PGF_{2\alpha}$ predominate with only small amounts of TXB_2 and PGI_2, while in the myometrium, conversion of arachidonic acid produces mainly prostacyclin and thromboxanes [13, 14]. Prostaglandin E_2 is a potent platelet disperser and vasodilator, while $PGF_{2\alpha}$ is a mediator and potentiator of pain sensation and a strong stimulator of smooth muscle contraction. Prostaglandin production in the uterus increases under the influence of estrogen, reaching a peak at, or soon after, the start of menstruation. Progesterone appears to inhibit prostaglandin synthesis until levels begin to fall just before menstruation [15]. Prostaglandin synthesis in the endometrium of the late secretory phase increases threefold over those of the proliferative phase. Data supports the assertion that it is $PGF_{2\alpha}$ and PGE_2 that are responsible for the vasospasm of the spiral arteries that typify the start of menstruation [16].

Once menstruation begins, the necrosis of endometrial cells provides increased substrate for the synthesis process when phospholipase A_2 converts the phospholipids of sloughed cell membranes into arachidonic acid. Both PGE_2 and $PGF_{2\alpha}$ concentrations are higher in the menstrual fluid of women with dysmenorrhea than in women with painless periods [17]: The highest concentrations of $PGF_{2\alpha}$ and PGE_2 are found in dysmenorrheic women during the first day of menstrual flow. In studies of non-dysmenorrheic women, the amount of $PGF_{2\alpha}$ and PGE_2 collected from menstrual fluid over 2 h correlated directly with total menstrual blood loss [18]. Indeed, in women diagnosed with menorrhagia, PGE_2 synthesis and the number of PGE-binding sites are greater in uterine tissues compared with those of normal women, and correlate directly with menstrual blood loss [19–22]. Synthesis of PGI_2 and nitric oxide are also high in menstrual blood collected from endometrium of women presenting with heavy menstrual bleeding [23, 24]. This suggests that the degree or duration of menstrual bleeding in women with menorrhagia may be extended by an increase in these vasodilatory factors.

The uterine activity induced by $PGF_{2\alpha}$ in patients with primary dysmenorrhea can be striking. During normal menstruation, contractions of 50–80 mmHg, lasting 15–30 s, are common and assist in the expulsion of blood and shed endometrial tissues. These contractions generally occur with a frequency of 1–4 contractions in 10 min. Resting pressure in the uterus is generally low and in the range of 5–15 mmHg. In women with dysmenorrhea, contractions may have peak pressure in excess of 400 mmHg, last longer than 90 s, and have less than 15 s of rest at a baseline pressure sometimes as high as 80–100 mmHg [25] (Fig. 6.10).

Uterine activity of this magnitude easily exceeds perfusion pressure, potentially causing significant ischemia, a potential source for nociceptive pain signals. The exact mechanism that creates the sensation of pain in dysmenorrhea is unknown. Studies show a strong correlation between pain and pain relief and the parameters

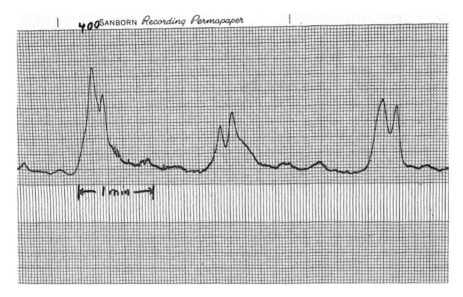

Fig. 6.10 An example of intrauterine pressures recorded from a young woman with dysmenorrhea during the first few hours of menstrual flow. The pressure scale is from 0 to 400 mmHg in this recording. Peak pressures seen here are as high as 350 mmHg, with resting pressure of 40 mmHg or higher. The pain reported by the patient was only "moderate" as compared to other periods

of uterine work, maximal pressures, frequency and quality of contractions, rate of pressure change, and the quality of "rest" between uterine contractions [25]. With the exception of rate of change, these parameters all have intuitive bearing on perfusion and ischemia.

In many nonhuman species, prostaglandin $F_{2\alpha}$ acts on the corpus luteum to cause luteolysis, forming a corpus albicans and stopping the production of progesterone. The action of $PGF_{2\alpha}$ is dependent on the number of G receptors on the corpus luteum membrane, through a general and transient block of the luteal adenylate cyclase system [26]. A positive feedback loop between endometrial $PGF_{2\alpha}$ and luteal oxytocin is responsible for completion of luteolysis [27].

In humans, there appears to be a luteotropic function of PGE_2 in regulation of the corpus luteum. Studies suggest that the main prostaglandin produced in human luteal tissue changes from PGE_2 to $PGF_{2\alpha}$ during the maturation and regression of the corpus luteum, and the loss of PGE_2 is more important than the effects of $PGF_{2\alpha}$ during luteolysis in women [28].

Studies show that the concentrations of prostaglandins are higher in the menstrual blood of women with endometriosis [29]. In parallel with dysmenorrhea studies, Bulletti et al. found that frequency, amplitude, and basal pressure tone of uterine contractions in women with endometriosis were higher than in those without [30].

Across all species, the processes that culminate in labor are characterized by an increased synthesis of prostaglandins by gestational tissues [31]. In humans, the administration of PGE_2 or $PGF_{2\alpha}$ will induce abortion in early pregnancy and labor at term. The fetal membranes and placenta are significant sources of prostaglandin synthesis, acting on increased levels of arachidonic acid present in amniotic fluid, especially during labor [32]. It is well established that $PGF_{2\alpha}$ is important in the softening of the cervix at term and there is evidence of altered production of prostaglandins in dysfunctional labor [33].

Key Points

- Prostaglandins are critical regulatory molecules that act on neighboring cells (paracrine function) or within the cells where they are made (autocrine function).
- All prostanoids are made as needed and are not stored.
- The common substrate for the production of prostanoids is arachidonic acid that is derived mainly from dietary sources and stored in cell membranes.
- Prostaglandin E_2 and $F_{2\alpha}$ are produced from PGG_2 and PGH_2, which are under the synthetic control of cyclooxygenase.
- Cyclooxygenase exists in two main isoforms, COX-1 and COX-2.
- In the uterus, it is prostaglandin E_2 and $F_{2\alpha}$ that are most important in the creation of menorrhagia and dysmenorrhea (respectively).

References

1. Blackwell CJ, Carnuccio R, DiRosa M, Flower RJ, Parente L, Persico P. Macrocortin: a polypeptide causing the anti-phospholipase effects of glucocorticoids. Nature. 1980;287:147–9.
2. Samitas K, Chorianopoulos D, Vittorakis S, et al. Exhaled cysteinyl-leukotrienes and 8-isoprostane in patients with asthma and their relation to clinical severity. Respir Med. 2009;103(5):750–6.
3. Spector AA, Fang X, Snyder GD, Weintraub NL. Epoxyeicosatrienoic acids (EETs): metabolism and biochemical function. Prog Lipid Res. 2004;43(1):55–90.
4. Jiang JG, Chen CL, Card JW, et al. Cytochrome P450 2J2 promotes the neoplastic phenotype of carcinoma cells and is up-regulated in human tumors. Cancer Res. 2005;65(11):4707–15.
5. Wagner K, Vito S, Inceoglu B, Hammock BD. The role of long chain fatty acids and their epoxide metabolites in nociceptive signaling. Prostaglandins Other Lipid Mediat. 2014;113–115:2–12.
6. Minami T, Nakano H, Kobayashi T, et al. Characterization of EP receptor subtypes responsible for prostaglandin E2-induced pain responses by use of EP1 and EP3 receptor knockout mice. Br J Pharmacol. 2001;133:438–44.
7. Foote EB. Plain home talk about the human system—the habits of men and women—the cause and prevention of disease--our sexual relations and social natures. New York: Murray Hill Publishing Company; 1896. p. 405.
8. Kawabata A. Prostaglandin E2 and pain—an update. Biol Pharm Bull. 2011;34(8):1170–3.
9. Chan BS, Satriano JA, Pucci M, Schuster VL. Mechanism of prostaglandin E2 transport across the plasma membrane of HeLa cells and Xenopus oocytes expressing the prostaglandin transporter "PGT". J Biol Chem. 1998;273:6689–97.
10. Ishihara O, Sullivan MH, Elder MG. Differences of metabolism of prostaglandin E2 and F2 alpha by decidual stromal cells and macrophages in culture. Eicosanoids. 1991;4(4):203–7.
11. Hitomi M, Shu J, Strom D, Hiebert SW, Harter ML, Stacey DW. Prostaglandin A2 blocks the activation of G1 phase cyclin-dependent kinase without altering mitogen-activated protein kinase stimulation. J Biol Chem. 1996;271(16):9376–83.

12. Lin S, Wang W, Wilson GM, et al. Down-regulation of cyclin D1 expression by prostaglandin A(2) is mediated by enhanced cyclin D1 mRNA turnover. Mol Cell Biol. 2000;20(21): 7903–13.

13. Moonen P, Klok G, Kierse MJNC. Immunohistochemical localization of prostaglandin endoperoxide synthase and prostacyclin synthase in pregnant human myometrium. Eur J Obstet Gynecol Reprod Biol. 1985;19:151–8.

14. Abel MH, Kelly RW. Differential production of prostaglandins within the human uterus. Prostaglandins. 1979;18:821–8.

15. Schatz F, Markiewicz I, Schatz F, Hirata F. *In vitro* effects of ovarian steroids on prostaglandin output by human endometrium and endometrial epithelial cells. J Clin Endocrinol Metab. 1985;61:361–7.

16. Abel MH, Kelly RW. Metabolism of prostaglandins by the non-pregnant human uterus. J Clin Endocrinol Metab. 1983;56:678–85.

17. Rees MC. Heavy painful periods. Ballieres Clin Obstet Gynacol. 1989;3:341–56.

18. Rees MC, Anderson AB, Demers LM, Turnbull AC. Prostaglandins in menstrual fluid in menorrhagia and dysmenorrhoea. Br J Obstet Gynaecol. 1984;91(7):673–80.

19. Smith SK, Abel MH, Kelly RW, Baird DT. Prostaglandin synthesis in the endometrium of women with ovular dysfunctional uterine bleeding. Br J Obstet Gynaecol. 1981;88(4): 434–42.

20. Hofmann GE, Rao CV, Barrows GH, Sanfilippo JS. Topography of human uterine prostaglandin E and F2 alpha receptors and their profiles during pathological states. J Clin Endocrinol Metab. 1983;57(2):360–6.

21. Rees MC, Anderson AB, Demers LM, Turnbull AC. Endometrial and myometrial prostaglandin release during the menstrual cycle in relation to menstrual blood loss. J Clin Endocrinol Metab. 1984;58(5):813–8.

22. Adelantado JM, López Bernal A, Turnbull AC. Increased uterine prostaglandin E receptors in menorrhagic women. Br J Obstet Gynaecol. 1988;95(2):162–5.

23. Smith SK, Abel MH, Kelly RW, Baird DT. A role for prostacyclin (PGi2) in excessive menstrual bleeding. Lancet. 1981;1(8219):522–4.

24. Mäkäräinen L, Ylikorkala O. Primary and myoma-associated menorrhagia: role of prostaglandins and effects of ibuprofen. Br J Obstet Gynaecol. 1986;93(9):974–8.

25. Smith RP, Powell JR. Simultaneous objective and subjective evaluation of meclofenamate sodium in the treatment of primary dysmenorrhea. Am J Obstet Gynecol. 1987;157(3):611–6.

26. Norjavaara E, Rosberg S. Mechanism of action of prostaglandin F2 alpha-induced luteolysis: evidence for a rapid effect on the guanine nucleotide binding regulatory component of adenylate cyclase in rat luteal tissue. Mol Cell Endocrinol. 1986;48(2–3):97–104.

27. Fuchs AR. Prostaglandin F2 alpha and oxytocin interactions in ovarian and uterine function. J Steroid Biochem. 1987;27(4–6):1073–80.

28. Nio-Kobayashi J, Kudo M, Sakuragi N, Iwanaga T, Duncan WC. Loss of luteotropic prostaglandin E plays an important role in the regulation of luteolysis in women. Mol Hum Reprod. 2017;23(5):271–81.

29. Karck U, Reister F, Schäfer W, Zahrandnik HP, Breckwoldt M. PGE2 and PGF2 alpha release by human peritoneal macrophages in endometriosis. Prostaglandins. 1996;51:49–60.

30. Bulletti C, De Ziegler D, Polli V, Del Ferro E, Palini S, Flamigni C. Characteristics of uterine contractility during menses in women with mild to moderate endometriosis. Fertile Steril. 2002;77:1156–61.

31. Rice GE. Labour: a process dependent upon prostaglandin G/H synthase. Reprod Fertil Dev. 1990;2:523–33.

32. Ogburn PL Jr, Brenner WE, Dingfelder JR, et al. Arachidonic acid's role in the pathology and physiology of pregnancy and labor. Prog Lipid Res. 1981;20:243–6.

33. Norman RJ, Reddi K. Prostaglandins in dysfunctional labor; evidence for altered production of prostaglandin $F_{2\alpha}$. Reprod Fertil Dev. 1990;2:563–74.

Additional Resources

Excellent overviews of prostaglandin metabolism, function, and their roles in dysmenorrhea and heavy menstrual bleeding can be found in:

Bailey JM, editor. Prostaglandins, leukotrienes, lipoxins and PAF: mechanism of action, molecular biology, and clinical applications. New York and London: Plenum Press; 1991.

Duckitt K. Menorrhagia. BMJ Clin Evid .2015 Sep 18;2015.

Duckitt K, Collins S. Menorrhagia. BMJ Clin Evid. 2012 Jan 18;2012.

Fraser IS. Prostaglandins, prostaglandin inhibitors and their roles in gynaecological disorders. Baillieres Clin Obstet Gynaecol. 1992;6(4):829–57.

Karim SMM, editor. The prostaglandins. New York: Wiley-Interscience; 1972.

Nygren KG, Rybo G. Prostaglandins and menorrhagia. Acta Obstet Gynecol Scand Suppl. 1983;113:101–3.

Ramwell PW, Foegh M, Loeb R, Leovey EM. Synthesis and metabolism of prostaglandins, prostacyclin, and thromboxanes: the arachidonic acid cascade. Semin Perinatol. 1980;4(1):3–13.

Smith WM. Prostanoid biosynthesis and mechanisms of action. Am J Phys. 1992;263(2 Pt 2):F181–91.

Smyth EM, Grosser T, Wang M, Yu Y, FitzGerald GA. Prostanoids in health and disease. J Lipid Res. 2009;50(Suppl):S423–8.

Chapter 7
The Inhibition of Prostaglandin Formation

7.1 Topic Overview

The primary therapeutic modality for patients with primary dysmenorrhea and heavy menstrual bleeding is the nonsteroidal anti-inflammatory drugs (NSAIDs). These agents act primarily to block the formation of the prostaglandins responsible for the symptoms. As noted in the previous chapter, the two prostaglandins responsible, PGE_2 and $PGF_{2\alpha}$, are both made from arachidonic acid through the enzymatic action of cyclooxygenases. Found in two main isoforms, COX-1 and COX-2, the characteristics of these two enzymes allow for specific and effective inhibition of their function. Understanding how this occurs, and the differences between agents that inhibit these enzymes, allows the clinician to better understand and choose effective therapy.

7.2 Cyclooxygenase Isoforms

Cyclooxygenase, officially known as prostaglandin-endoperoxide synthase (PTGS), is actually a family of at least three isoforms that are responsible for the metabolic conversion of arachidonic acid into prostanoids. Cyclooxygenase-1 (COX-1) is constitutively produced in most cells, while COX-2 synthesis is induced by stimuli such as interleukin-1, and reduced by glucocorticoids [1]. This suppression of COX expression by glucocorticoids is specific to COX-2.

The third isoform, COX-3, is a variant of COX-1 found in highest concentrations in the cerebral cortex and heart tissue [2]. Some studies have demonstrated that acetaminophen produces an analgesic and antipyretic effect in mice by inhibiting COX-3 in the brain, decreasing levels of brain PGE_2 [3]. Its role in humans remains to be more fully elucidated.

© Springer International Publishing AG 2018
R.P. Smith, *Dysmenorrhea and Menorrhagia*,
https://doi.org/10.1007/978-3-319-71964-1_7

Fig. 7.1 A schematic representation of COX-1 and COX-2 showing the wider access to the active enzymatic site and the side pocket characteristic of COX-2

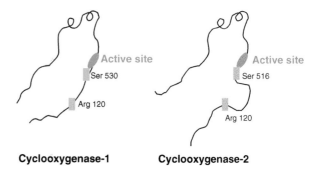

Cyclooxygenase-1   **Cyclooxygenase-2**

Cyclooxygenase-1 and COX-2, homodimers of 576 and 581 amino acids, respectively, have similar molecular weights (approximately 70 and 72 kDa, respectively), have approximately 61% amino acid sequence homology, and have nearly identical catalytic sites. The greatest difference between the two forms is the substitution of isoleucine at position 523 in COX-1 with valine in COX-2. This results in a 17% wider channel leading to the active site and a side pocket that increases volume by additional 8%. The smaller valine molecule in COX-2 allows access to a hydrophobic side pocket in the enzyme, which isoleucine sterically hinders. When the cellular concentrations of arachidonic acid are high, metabolism by COX-1 predominates, while at low concentrations, COX-2 reactions predominate [4] (Fig. 7.1).

Each COX isozyme contains three major domains: an N-terminal epidermal growth factor domain, a helical membrane-binding domain, and a large catalytic domain at the C-terminus, which contains two main active sites[1] on either side of a heme prosthetic group. The membrane-binding domain contains four helices, which surround the opening where fatty acids and NSAIDs enter into the core of the globular portion of the protein. The upper portion of the catalytic domain at the C-terminus makes up the cyclooxygenase active site that binds these fatty acids and NSAIDs. The cleft is hydrophobic, and in the absence of an inhibitor, arachidonic acid diffuses into the channel and bonds with arginine at position 120 (Arg_{120}) and serine at position 530 (Ser_{530}) [6]. An electron transfer from tyrosine (Tyr_{385} in COX-1) to an oxidized heme moiety bound to the enzyme begins the conversion of arachidonic acid to prostaglandin G [7] (Fig. 7.2).

In COX-1 and COX-2, there are distinct cyclooxygenase and hydroperoxidase active sites. Imidazole groups (His_{309} and His_{388}) occupy the axial positons of the heme moiety if no peroxide is present (when present, in sixth position as shown in

---

[1] There are actually 19 cyclooxygenase active site residues that are predicted to make a total of 50 contacts with the substrate. These fall into five functional categories: those directly involved in hydrogen abstraction from C-13 of arachidonate (Tyr_{385}), residues essential for positioning C-13 of arachidonate for hydrogen abstraction (Gly_{533} and Tyr_{348}), residues critical for high-affinity arachidonate binding (Arg_{120}), residues critical for positioning arachidonate in a conformation so that the molecule is optimally arranged to yield PGG_2 versus monohydroperoxy acid products (Val_{349}, Trp_{387}, and Leu_{534}), and all other active residues [5].

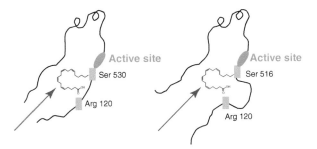

Fig. 7.2 Arachidonic acid enters the cleft in the COX enzyme and bonds to arginine at position 120 and serine at position 530 (Ser_{516} in COX-2). Electron transfer from tyrosine at location 385 initiates the cyclooxygenase reaction

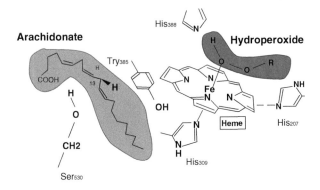

Fig. 7.3 A schematic representation of the arachidonic acid binding site in cyclooxygenase

the figure). Tyr_{385} is positioned between the heme/hydroperoxidase and arachidonate binding sites and is responsible for the oxygen transfer noted above [5] (Fig. 7.3).

In the cyclooxygenase reaction, two molecules of oxygen are added to arachidonic acid to form a bicyclic endoperoxide with a further hydroperoxy group in position 15, forming PGG_2. The first reaction occurs within the cleft at the center of the enzyme, before the hydroperoxide intermediate is transferred to the heme-containing site on the surface of the enzyme. Here it is reduced by a peroxidase to form prostaglandin PGH_2.

7.3   Inhibiting Cyclooxygenase Formation and Function

In 1971, Sir John Vane proposed that the main mechanism of action of nonsteroidal anti-inflammatory drugs was the inhibition of prostaglandin production [8]. The classical cyclooxygenase inhibitors are not selective and inhibit all forms of the enzyme to varying extents. The resulting inhibition of prostaglandin and thromboxane synthesis has the effect of reducing inflammation and is antipyretic, antithrombotic, and analgesic.

The most frequent adverse effect of NSAIDs is irritation of the gastric lining because prostaglandins normally have a protective role in the stomach, where endogenous prostaglandins modulate acid secretion by blocking the histamine-stimulated increase in cyclic AMP within the parietal cell, in response to gastric pH. The major prostaglandins produced by the gastric mucosa are PGE_2 and PGI_2, with lesser amounts of $PGF_{2\alpha}$ and PGD_2 also found. Mucus and bicarbonate secretion by both the stomach and duodenum are also influenced by these endogenous prostaglandins. Gaseous mediators (nitric oxide and hydrogen sulfide) and neuropeptides (calcitonin gene-related peptide, CGRP) also play a role in protecting the stomach from injury.

The inhibition of cyclooxygenase can happen reversibly or irreversibly, though most inhibitors do so reversibly through competition with the lipid substrate for the active binding site. This occurs when the blocking molecule enters the enzymatic cleft and bonds with one or both binding sites, Arg_{120} or Ser_{530}, preventing access by the normal lipid substrate. Because of the small size and often linear shape of the non-specific COX inhibitors, the blocking molecules can enter the cleft of either isoform (Fig. 7.4).

In the case of aspirin (acetylsalicylic acid), the inhibition is irreversible because aspirin permanently acetylates the enzymatically active site by covalently attaching an acetyl group to the hydroxyl of the Ser_{530} residue in COX-1 (Ser_{516} in COX-2) [9], which is juxtaposed to Arg_{120}. Arginine-120 is part of a hydrogen-bonding network with Glu_{524} and Tyr_{355}, which stabilizes substrate/inhibitor interactions and closes off the upper part of the cyclooxygenase active site from the larger opening at the base of the cleft. Acetylation of the enzyme by aspirin places a bulky substituent on the serine oxygen that inhibits binding of arachidonic acid [10]. However, the slightly larger active site of COX-2 can allow some arachidonic acid to move past the aspirin molecule inactivating COX-2 and become converted to 15-R-hydroperoxyeicosatetraenoic acid (HETE) and other lipoxins [11]. Aspirin also diverts the COX-2 enzymatic activity toward the synthesis of precursors of lipoxin A_4, a potent anti-inflammatory lipid [12] (Fig. 7.5).

As noted above, non-specific COX inhibitors are usually small, often linear molecules that fit easily into the enzymatic cleft. Selective COX-2 inhibitors are generally made up of bulkier, three-ring structures with a side chain that is too big to enter

Fig. 7.4 The relatively small molecular size of non-specific nonsteroidal anti-inflammatory agents, such as aspirin (shown), gives them free access to the COX-1 and COX-2 active sites

acetylsalicylic acid

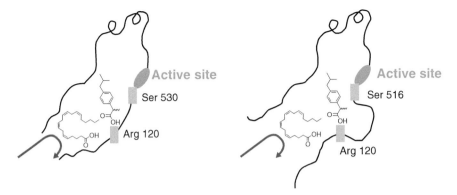

Fig. 7.5 Inhibition of cyclooxygenase occurs when an inhibitor occupies the normal lipid-binding site, preventing the normal ligand from accessing the binding and active sites. The reversible inhibition of COX-1 and COX-2 metabolism of arachidonic acid by ibuprofen is schematically shown

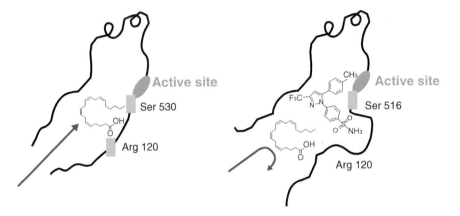

Fig. 7.6 Selective COX-2 inhibitors, such as celecoxib (schematically shown), are too large to fit into the smaller COX-1 cleft, allowing COX-1 to continue to function

the smaller cleft of COX-1. The side pocket formed because of the substitution of the smaller valine in COX-2 allows the accommodation of these larger, selective inhibitors that cannot fit into the COX-1 structure (Fig. 7.6).

7.4   Nonsteroidal Anti-inflammatory Drug Families

A large number of pharmaceutical and naturally occurring substances can inhibit the production, or in a few cases the actions, of prostaglandins. Broadly referred to as nonsteroidal anti-inflammatory drugs, these drugs may be grouped into

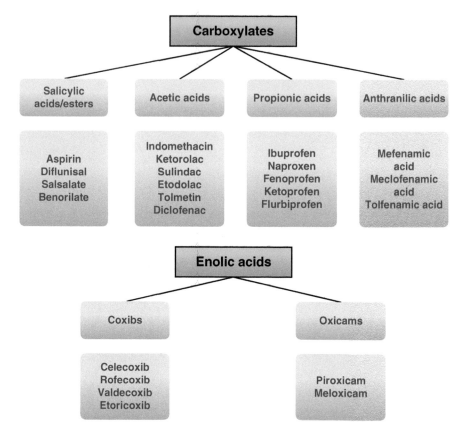

Fig. 7.7 Nonsteroidal anti-inflammatory drugs may be classified by their chemical derivation. Representative members of each class are shown

categories based upon their shared chemistry, their mechanism of action, or their degree of cyclooxygenase isoform specificity. Because, clinically, drugs that are chemically related often perform similarly, it is that classification that will be used here (Fig. 7.7).

Arguably, the oldest NSAID is acetylsalicylic acid. Originally trademarked and marketed by the Bayer corporation as Aspirin™, anti-German sentiment during World War I and the company's own failure to use the name in its early advertising resulted in the trademark being lost in 1918, making "aspirin" the generic term in this and many other countries. Derived from salicylic acid, the drugs in this class are generally not used in the treatment of dysmenorrhea and heavy menstrual bleeding. Aspirin has greater effect on COX function than do the other members of this class—much of their therapeutic effects are thought to occur in other means. For example, salicylic acid works not by direct inhibition of COX but instead by suppression of the expression of the enzyme through an unknown mechanism [13] (Fig. 7.8).

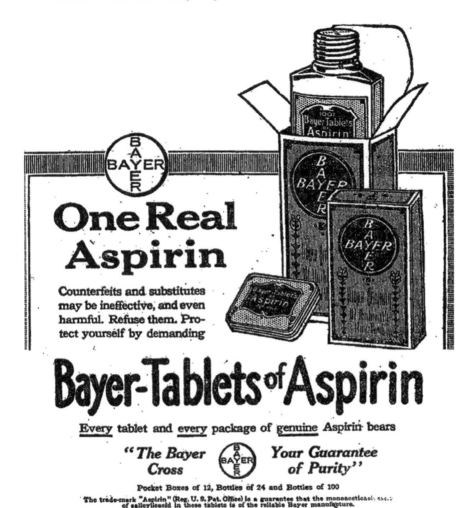

Fig. 7.8 One of the early US advertisements for Bayer Aspirin as published in the *New York Times*, February 19, 1917, p. 6

Acetic acid derivatives, such as indomethacin, were actually some of the first NSAIDs to show efficacy in dysmenorrhea, when young women with juvenile rheumatoid arthritis noticed menstrual benefit in addition to the effect on their joints. Indomethacin and other drugs in this group have a narrow therapeutic range between efficacy and toxicity, have a gradual onset of action, and reach peak effect (and blood levels) after repeated doses. Because of the latter, these drugs are better suited to long-term treatment settings, such as in arthritis. Many of the drugs in the class, such as indomethacin and ketorolac, have significant renal effects, which can cause edema and lithium toxicity. While indomethacin is nonselective, diclofenac and etodolac can inhibit COX-1 but appear to have a predilection for COX-2 [14].

Fig. 7.9 Chemically
similar, the two most
commonly used propionic
acid derivatives are
ibuprofen and naproxen

Ibuprofen   Naproxen
(Motrin)   (Aleve)

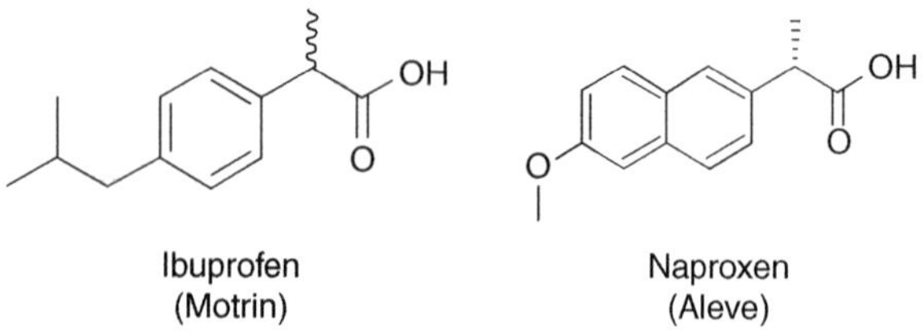

Diclofenac is perhaps the most potent of all the NSAIDs, requiring a very small dose to achieve therapeutic action [15], but its use has been associated with rare cases of Stevens-Johnson syndrome [16]. Despite potency, with efficacy that is comparable to other agents, increased costs, and the risk of major side effects, diclofenac is seldom used for the treatment of dysmenorrhea or heavy menstrual bleeding. The use of diclofenac as a veterinary pain reliever has been banned in most of the Indian subcontinent because of its renal toxicity, which can rapidly kill scavenging birds that eat dead animals. This came to the attention of conservationist in the 1990s, when there was a 99% decline of the population of white-rumped vulture (*Gyps bengalensis*), an Old World vulture native to South and Southeast Asia [17].

The 2-arylpropionic acid family of drugs are the most widely used over-the-counter NSAIDs, with ibuprofen and naproxen leading the market. Larger than the acetic acid derivatives and smaller than the fatty acids, this class of relatively mid-sized molecules act as non-specific COX inhibitors. Many of the forms unfamiliar to US prescribers are pro-drugs that undergo metabolism into their active form, most of which are similar to ibuprofen. Naproxen is associated with the smallest overall cardiovascular risks of the commonly used NSAIDs [18, 19]. In clinical use, the sodium salt is more quickly absorbed than the naproxen base (Fig. 7.9).

The anthranilic acid derivatives (fenamates) are less frequently used but highly effective nonselective COX inhibitors. A second mode of action has been demonstrated for fenamates, such as sodium meclofenamate and mefenamic acid, which inhibit the binding of PGE_2 to its receptor in addition to reducing prostaglandin synthesis [20]. Studies have indicated that these agents can be highly effective in blocking the excessive uterine activity of dysmenorrhea [21]. Higher costs and a higher incidence of gastrointestinal side effects have limited the use of these agents.

When the coxib family of NSAIDs was first introduced, they were seen as a major step forward, offering the hope of blocking the adverse impact of COX-2 while leaving the maintenance functions of COX-1 intact. Unfortunately, as experience with them expanded and our understanding of the complex roles of COX-1 and COX-2 became more nuanced, it became apparent that these agents were associated with an almost 40% increase in incidence of major vascular events, including nonfatal myocardial infarction, nonfatal stroke, or death from a blood vessel-related cause [19]. This, combined with a high level of gastrointestinal complications, resulted in withdrawal of rofecoxib and valdecoxib (Vioxx and Bextra) from the market in the United States and the addition of black box warnings for celecoxib

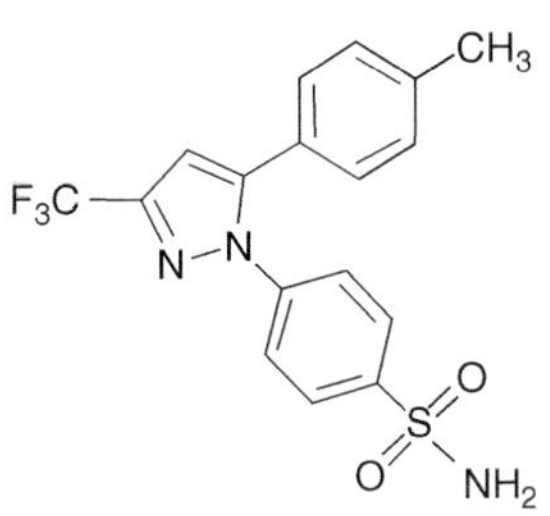

**Celecoxib
(Celebrex)**

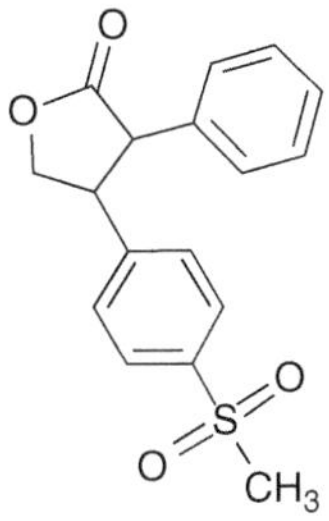

**Rofecoxib
(Vioxx)***

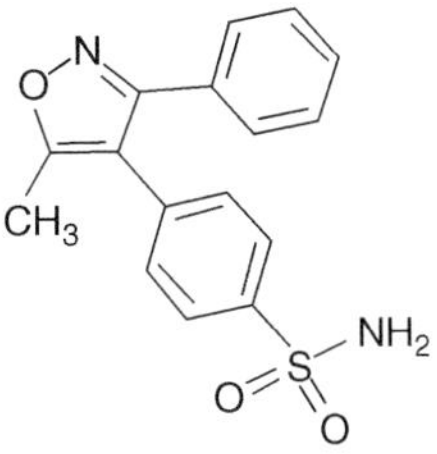

**Valdecoxib
(Bextra)***

*Withdrawn 2004   *Withdrawn 2005

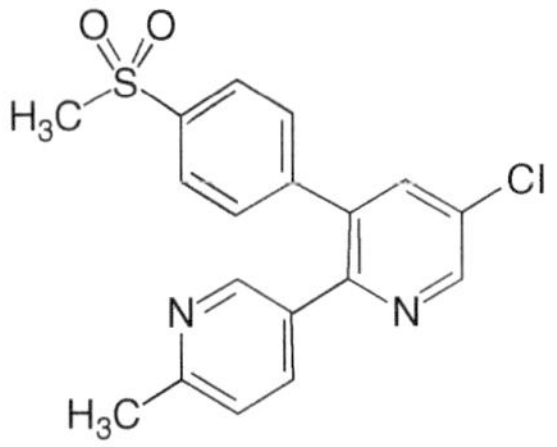

**Etoricoxib†
(Arcoxia)**

†Not available in the U.S.

Fig. 7.10 With the exception of celecoxib, the majority of the bulkier inhibitors that preferentially affected COX-2 have been withdrawn from the US market

(Celebrex). As analgesics, drugs in this class are comparable to ibuprofen in efficacy [22] with some exceptions [23]. Some of the drugs in this class have been associated with Stevens-Johnson syndrome (Fig. 7.10).

Key Points
- Cyclooxygenase exists in two isoforms that have slight differences in their structure and function that can be exploited therapeutically.
- Cyclooxygenase-2 has a wider cleft and a bulge near the catalytic site that allows larger inhibitory molecules selective access.
- Selective COX-2 inhibitors generally have a less linear molecular structure than do the nonselective agents.
- Nonsteroidal anti-inflammatory drugs generally fall into two broad chemical groups: carboxylates and enolic acid derivatives.
- In general, drugs from the same chemical class will have very similar therapeutic profiles.

References

1. Fu J, Masferrer J, Seibert K, Raz A, Needleman P. The induction and suppression of prosta-glandin H2 synthase (cyclooxygenase) in human monocytes. J Clin Invest. 1990;86:16737–40.
2. Chandrasekharan NV, Dai H, Roos LT, et al. COX-3, a cyclooxygenase-1 variant inhibited by acetaminophen and other analgesic/antipyretic drugs: cloning, structure, and expression. Proc Natl Acad Sci U S A. 2002;99:13926–31.
3. Botting R, Ayoub SS. COX-3 and the mechanism of action of paracetamol/acetaminophen. Prostaglandins Leukot Essent Fatty Acids. 2005;72:85–7.
4. Shitashige M, Morita I, Murota S. Different substrate utilization between prostaglandin endo-peroxide H synthase-1 and-2 in NIH3T3 fibroblasts. Biochim Biophys Acta. 1998;1389:57–66.
5. Thuresson ED, Lakkides KM, Rieke CJ, et al. Prostaglandin Endoperoxide H Synthase-1: the functions of cyclooxygenase active site residues in the binding, positioning, and oxygenation of arachidonic acid. J Biol Chem. 2001;276(13):10347–59.
6. Marnett LJ, Rowlinson SW, Goodwin DC, Kalgutkar AS, Lanzo CA. Arachidonic acid oxy-genation by COX- and COX-2. J Biol Chem. 1999;274(33):22903–6.
7. Tsai A-L, Kulmacz RJ, Palmer G. Spectroscopic evidence for reaction of prostaglandin H synthase-1 tyrosyl radical with arachidonic acid. J Biol Chem. 1995;270(18):10503–8.
8. Vane JR. Inhibition of prostaglandin synthesis as a mechanism of action for aspirin-like drugs. Nat New Biol. 1971;231:232–5.
9. Roth GJ, Majerus PW. The mechanism of the effect of Aspirin on human platelets: 1. Acetylation of a particulate fraction protein. J Clin Invest. 1975;56:624–32.
10. De Witt FL, El-Harith EA, Kraemer SA, et al. The Aspirin and heme-binding sites of ovine and murine prostaglandin endoperoxide synthases. J Biol Chem. 1990;265:5192–8.
11. Vane JR, Bakhle YS, Botting RM. Cyclooxygenases 1 and 2. Annu Rev Pharmacol Toxicol. 1998;38:97–120.
12. Serhan CN, Clish CB, Brannon J, Colgan SP, Chiang N, Gronert K. Novel functional sets of lipid-derived mediators with anti-inflammatory actions generated from omega-3 fatty acids via cyclooxygenase 2-nonsteroidal anti-inflammatory drugs and transcellular processing. J Exp Med. 2000;192:1197–204.
13. Xu X-M, Sansores-Garcia L, Chen X-M, Matijevic-Aleksic N, Du M, Wu KK. Suppression of inducible cyclooxygenases-2 gene transcription by aspirin and sodium salicylate. Proc Natl Acad Sci U S A. 1999;96:5292–7.
14. Ku EC, Lee W, Kothari HV, Scholer DW. Effect of diclofenac sodium on the arachidonic acid cascade. Am J Med. 1986;80:18–23.
15. Scholer DW. Pharmacology of diclofenac sodium. Am J Med. 1986;80:34–8.
16. Roujeau J-C, Kelly JP, Naldi L, et al. Medication use and the risk of Stevens-Johnson syn-drome or toxic epidermal necrolysis. N Engl J Med. 1995;333(1):1600–7.
17. Oaks JL, Gilbert M, Virani MZ, et al. Diclofenac residues as the cause of vulture population decline in Pakistan. Nature. 2004;427:630–3.
18. Trelle S, Reichenbach S, Wandel S, et al. Cardiovascular safety of non-steroidal anti-inflammatory drugs: network meta-analysis. BMJ. 2011;342:c7086.
19. Bhala N, Emberson J, Merhi A, et al. Vascular and upper gastrointestinal effects of non-steroidal anti-inflammatory drugs: meta-analyses of individual participant data from random-ized trials. Lancet. 2013;382(9894):769–79.
20. Rees MC, Cañete-Solér R, López Bernal A, Turnbull AC. Effect of fenamates on prostaglandin E receptor binding. Lancet. 1988;2(8610):541–2.
21. Smith RP, Powell JR. Intrauterine pressure changes during mefenamic acid treatment of pri-mary spasmodic dysmenorrhea. Am J Obstet Gynecol. 1982;143:286–92.
22. Derry S, Moore RA. Single dose oral celecoxib for acute postoperative pain in adults. Cochrane Database Syst Rev. 2013;(10):CD004233.
23. Clarke R, Derry S, Moore RA. Single dose oral etoricoxib for acute postoperative pain in adults. Cochrane Database Syst Rev. 20148;(5):CD004309.

Additional Resources

Good overviews of this topic can be found at:

Botting RM. Cyclooxygenase: past, present and future. A tribute to John R. Vane (1927–2004). J Therm Biol. 2006;31:208–19.

Copeland RA, Williams JM, Giannaras J, et al. Mechanism of selective inhibition of the inducible isoform of prostaglandidn G/H synthase. Proc Natl Acad Sci U S A. 1994;91:11202–6.

Grosser T, Ricciotti E, FitzGerald GA. The cardiovascular pharmacology of nonsteroidal anti-inflammatory drugs. Trends Pharmacol Sci. 2017 Jun 23. pii: S0165-6147(17)30116-5.

Kurumbail RG, Kiefer JR, Marnett LJ. Cyclooxygenase enzymes: catalysis and inhibition. Curr Opin Struct Biol. 2001;11:752–60.

Marnett LJ. Recent developments in cyclooxygenase inhibition. Prostaglandins Other Lipid Mediat. 2002;68–69:153–64.

Park JY, Pillinger MH, Abramson SB. Prostaglandin E_2 synthesis and secretion: the role of PGE2 synthases. Clin Immunol. 2006;119:229–40.

Picot D, Loll PJ, Garavito RM. The X-ray crystal structure of the membrane protein prostaglandin H2 synthase-1. Nature. 1994;367:243–9.

So O-Y, Scarafia LE, Mak AY, Callan OH, Swinnery DC. The dynamics of prostaglandin H synthases. J Biol Chem. 1998;273(10):5801–7.

Vitale P, Panella A, Scilimati A, Perrone MG. COX-1 inhibitors: beyond structure toward therapy. Med Res Rev. 2016;36(4):641–71.

Chapter 8
Establishing the Diagnosis

8.1 Topic Overview

As in most of medicine, effective treatment of a patient's concerns or symptoms demands an accurate diagnosis of the problem. Unfortunately, in the cases of painful or heavy menses, the process of establishing a diagnosis is not always straightforward. For women with painful menses, there is the non-specific nature of the symptoms, the variability of presentation, and the youth and sexual innocence of many of its sufferers; women who report heavy menstrual bleeding have no reliable index for measurement or comparison. In both cases, the actual symptoms often happen far from the clinical setting, physically or temporally. These challenges may be surmounted with a systematic approach to the diagnostic process, most of which is driven by a careful, thorough review of the patient's history. For this discussion, we will ignore situations in which the diagnostic process for symptoms of pain or heavy bleeding is trivial, such as following the placement of an intrauterine contraceptive device, subsequent to a prolonged period of amenorrhea as in anovulation or polycystic ovary syndrome, or iatrogenic interventions such as anticoagulation.

8.2 Dysmenorrhea

Because it is important to differentiate patients with primary dysmenorrhea from those with symptoms secondary to other processes, the accuracy of the diagnostic process will foretell the efficacy of the treatment. In a majority of instances, a careful history will lead the clinician in the correct direction, but there still remains a place for the physical examination, laboratory, and imaging for select patients.

© Springer International Publishing AG 2018
R.P. Smith, *Dysmenorrhea and Menorrhagia*,
https://doi.org/10.1007/978-3-319-71964-1_8

8.2.1   History

As it does throughout medicine, the patient's history forms the basis of diagnosis in the majority of cases of painful menstruation. The exploration of the patient's symptoms must be thorough and wide-ranging, yet detailed, if a correct diagnosis is to be determined. While much of the focus of the dialog will, perforce, be directed to the patient's pain experience, other aspects of the history must not be overlooked. For example, the incidence of both dysmenorrhea and menorrhagia are roughly twofold higher in women who have been the victims of sexual assault or abuse [1], so this history should always be a part of any exploration of painful or excessive menses. (The presence of such a history should not be used as an excuse to dismiss the physical ailments the patient is experiencing or to impute causation (Table 8.1).)

Recent studies have looked at factors associated with primary dysmenorrhea [2], but their findings have not added significantly to what have been the historically related features. As a result, the history should begin in the classic way as with any presenting complaint: What is the nature of the discomfort?; what is its location, intensity, and duration?; what are its associated symptoms?; what are the things that modify the pain (better or worse)?; when did it begin?; how did it evolve?; etc. Pain that began 6–12 months after menarche, has gradually become worse, and is described using an opening and closing fist held over the lower abdomen suggests primary dysmenorrhea. Pain that started in the late thirties and is associated with pelvic fullness and heavy menstrual flow suggests secondary dysmenorrhea, such as that found with uterine leiomyomata (Fig. 8.1).

The age of menarche should be documented, because the severity of dysmenorrhea symptoms positively correlates with early menarche, and with increased duration and amount of menstrual flow, in some studies [4]. A sexual history should be taken, and contraceptive use and parity should be explored, though the relationship with parity has been mixed. For example, regression analysis has suggested that age is a stronger risk factor than almost all other factors studied, including parity [5]. A 2006 study of almost 3700 patients did find improvement with vaginal delivery of

Table 8.1 Historical focus in evaluating painful menstrual periods

Background
Family, review of symptoms (including psychosocial, drug and tobacco use)
Menstrual history
Menarche, regularity, duration, flow, abnormal bleeding
Pain
Age at onset, character, location, radiation, associated symptoms, timing with period, evolution over time, prior treatment(s)
Associated symptoms
Gastrointestinal (function, pain, bleeding) Urologic (urgency, pain) Musculoskeletal
Gynecologic
Pregnancy, surgery, infection, dyspareunia

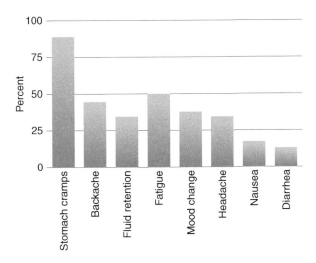

Fig. 8.1 The frequency of symptoms of primary dysmenorrhea reported by a group of 388 high school students in western Australia. Data from Hillen et al. [3]

first pregnancy. It also found that among nulliparous women, there were diminished symptoms in those who had more frequent intercourse and those who were older [6]. These results must be interpreted with care because of the study's use of a visual analog assessment of pain and the risk of recall bias over the 8-year study duration. Certainly, when dysmenorrhea occurs after pregnancy or delivery, a secondary cause for the symptoms should be sought. Worsening menstrual pain in the presence of involuntary infertility should suggest the possibility of endometriosis or pelvic scarring. A cross-sectional study found no difference in menstrual pain in women with and women without tubal sterilization [7], so the development of pain following a sterilization procedure suggests non-uterine causes.

A general review of symptoms and health history must be included. The frequency of dysmenorrhea is higher in smokers, those with menstrual irregularity, those who use drugs for menstrual regulation, and those having a family history of pain ($p < 0.05$ for each). In the same study, sleep quality was found to be poorer in students having a history of dysmenorrhea ($p < 0.05$) [8], though it must be recognized that it may be the cramping itself that is eroding sleep quality and not poor sleep bringing on menstrual dysfunction.

The patient's past experience with medications or other interventions, and the outcome of those attempts, should be explored. This can give insight into both past success and failures but also valuable hints about the underlying mechanisms of discomfort. However, it is important to recognize that in studies, 57% or more of those who self-medicated with over-the-counter treatments used subtherapeutic doses [9], only 54% of adolescents knew that certain medications could relieve menstrual cramps [10], and 27% of girls were unable to recognize any of three NSAID treatments for dysmenorrhea offered [3] (Fig. 8.2).

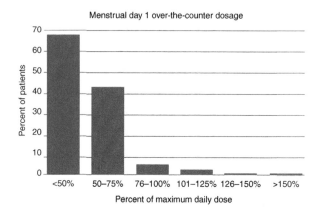

Fig. 8.2 Many patients take less than therapeutic doses of over-the-counter medications, as found in this group of 71 adolescents who reported self-medication. Data from O'Connell et al. [11]

Symptoms associated with the pain of menstruation may be pivotal in diagnosing cases of secondary dysmenorrhea. While gastrointestinal symptoms (cramps and diarrhea, predominately) are common with primary dysmenorrhea, the presence of symptoms outside the first day or two of menses would suggest conditions such as irritable or inflammatory bowel disease. Urinary frequency or urgency that increases during menses may foretell interstitial cystitis. Deep-thrust dyspareunia suggests pelvic scarring, endometriosis, or uterine leiomyomata, though it may also be present with interstitial cystitis and colonic pathologies. Patients who experience a sense of lower abdominal or pelvic fullness or heaviness that worsens with menses should be evaluated for uterine fibroids. Intermenstrual bleeding or bleeding with intercourse should suggest the possibility of a prolapsing polyp or myoma.

8.2.2   Physical Examination

In the majority of cases, the history will strongly suggest the cause of the patient's menstrual pain. In such cases, the physical examination, if done, should be targeted toward those probabilities or their mimics. In the absence of a history suspicious for secondary causes, the value of the pelvic examination is questionable. For example, pelvic examination has a 76% sensitivity, 74% specificity, 67% positive predictive value, and 81% negative predictive value for endometriosis [12]. Certainly, for teens and those who are virginal, unless significant pathology is deemed likely, empiric therapy without a pelvic examination seems justified (Fig. 8.3).

If performed, findings in those with secondary dysmenorrhea might include a fixed uterus, or reduced uterine mobility, adnexal masses, and uterosacral nodularity in patients with endometriosis, mucopurulent cervical discharge in those with chronic pelvic infections, and uterine enlargement or asymmetry in patients with adenomyosis [13]. Discomfort elicited by palpation of the base of the bladder is

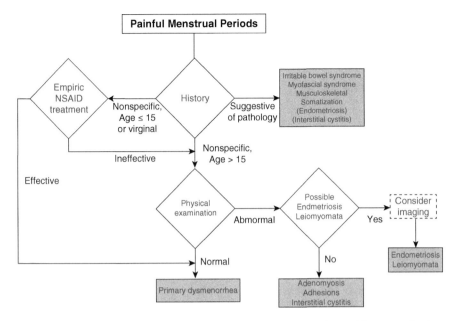

Fig. 8.3 One possible algorithm for establishing the diagnosis for patients with menstrual pain

common in patients with interstitial cystitis. Pain that results from abdominal wall palpation suggests myofascial syndrome or somatization.

One study advocated inspection of the tongue to diagnose primary dysmenorrhea [14], but this clearly requires additional evaluation and documentation before it can be recommended for wide-scale adoption. Another recent study reported using the traditional Korean physical assessment of "peripheral artery pulse wave analysis" to diagnose dysmenorrhea [15]. This, too, is likely not to become a mainstream tool in this country without wider study.

8.2.3 Laboratory and Imaging

Like the pelvic examination, laboratory and imaging modalities generally offer little assistance unless a very specific pathology is being considered and that pathology is one that can be differentiated by these tools. Transvaginal ultrasonography should be considered if secondary dysmenorrhea due to structural processes is likely [16], though it should be noted that the diagnosis of uterine leiomyomata remains one that can be established using only history and physical means and does not require confirmation with X-ray or ultrasonography. Ultrasonography has a reported 91% sensitivity and 98% specificity, a positive likelihood ratio of 30, and a negative likelihood ratio of 0.09 for detection of bowel endometriosis [17] and good accuracy for detection of ovarian endometriomas [12], but it is not infallible [18]. When such pathologies are being seriously considered, or initial treatments do not produce the expected results, direct investigation through diagnostic laparoscopy should be considered.

8.3 Menorrhagia

By the way the research description of menorrhagia was defined (population-based), only about 10% of menstruating women experience blood loss in excess of 80 mL per cycle. This level of blood loss was established as the threshold through the observations that anemia, without other apparent causes, was rarely seen with blood losses below 60–80 mL per cycle [19–21]. Because secondary menorrhagia is documented in roughly 50% of cases, the role of physical, laboratory, and imaging tools is much greater than in dysmenorrhea. Efforts to apply decision analysis techniques to define an optimal approach to the diagnosis of heavy menstrual bleeding have not yielded a clearly superior approach [22].

8.3.1 History

It has been reported that only about 25–40% of women with complaints of regular heavy menstrual bleeding have objective blood loss that exceed 80 mL [23–25]. In one study of women who rated their flow as very heavy, 25% had losses of less than 35 mL per cycle [26]. At the other extreme, some women do not consider heavy menstrual flow to be abnormal. This said, most clinicians feel that the patient's complaint of heavy bleeding is all that is required for the diagnosis of heavy menstrual bleeding. This is both pragmatic and functional. Certainly, such a presenting symptom must be taken seriously, explored, and addressed, since perception and inconvenience can be as much an intrusion into the patient's life as any pathologic threat might pose (Fig. 8.4).

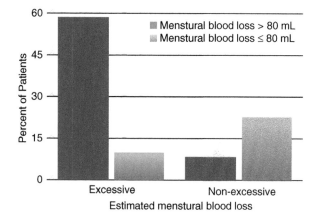

Fig. 8.4 Menstrual blood loss estimated by menstrual diary or visual assessment methods does not always reliably predict actual (measured) blood loss, as seen in this study of 648 bleeding episodes. Data from Schumacher et al. [27]

As with dysmenorrhea, a careful history will often suggest the possibility of underlying pathology (secondary menorrhagia). Once again, information about the onset of the symptoms, their evolution, the relationship to other events or symptoms, factors or treatments that alter the observation, and other information should be obtained. While the value has been questioned [23, 28], information about the menstrual hygiene methods used, frequency of change, duration of flow, and presence, number, and size of blood clots, is generally requested.

To assist this process, some have proposed tools to quantify blood loss outside of direct collection and measurement of menstrual hemoglobin. One such is that developed by Higham et al., the pictorial blood assessment chart (PBAC) [29]. This self-assessed chart consists of diagrams representing different soiled menstrual pads and tampons. Women are instructed to count their number of used pads or tampons each day and then record them by level of soiling. The PBAC tool was validated in adult women; a score greater than 100 in one menstrual cycle has a sensitivity and specificity of 80% for determining heavy blood loss [29]. A PBAC score of 150 points most accurately correlates with menstrual blood loss of ≥80 mL [30, 31]. Tools like this are not without limitations [30, 32], and other tools have also been proposed [33].

8.3.2   Physical Examination

Because the majority of abnormalities that are associated with heavy menstrual bleeding are found within the uterus, the physical examination in these women will be, at most, suggestive. For example, a diffusely enlarged, "woody" uterus is suggestive of adenomyosis, but it is far from diagnostic. A generous, but normal-sized, uterus could be caused by intracavitary pathologies but is often simply the result of childbearing. The notable exception is that of uterine leiomyomata, where myomas seldom exist in isolation and palpable myomas distorting the uterus are sufficient to establish a working diagnosis without further imaging. It should not be forgotten that by simple physical examination it is often possible to broadly rule out significant anemia or increase the suspicion that it may be present through inspection of the palm, nail beds, or sclera (Fig. 8.5).

8.3.3   Laboratory and Imaging

Based on the issues identified in the patient's history, the first priority may be the validation of the problem, even before a physical examination. A simple in-office assessment of hemoglobin or hematocrit may suffice in many instances, while in others a complete blood count with iron studies may better define iron status. Iron deficiency anemia develops in 21–67% percent of women with heavy menstrual bleeding [19, 20, 34]. A low ferritin level correctly predicts 60% of women with

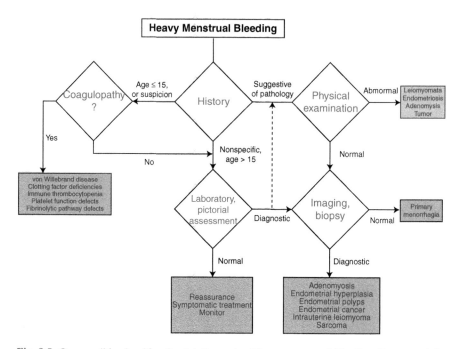

Fig. 8.5 One possible algorithm for the diagnosis of heavy menstrual bleeding. Because of the limited yield of the physical examination, its role is limited and variable. Similarly, laboratory assessments to establish the presence of iron deficiency anemia may or may not be needed in each case. Most of the decision points must be tempered by clinical judgment and needs of the individual patient

periods with measured losses of more than 80 mL per menstrual cycle. When combined with a history of changing a pad or tampon more than hourly, and passing clots larger than 1 in. diameter, prediction is enhanced [26]. It has been suggested that when anemia is not present, the patient should be requested to use one of the visual assessment tools to chart their blood loss before further diagnostic or therapeutic steps are taken [35].

Based upon suspicion, an evaluation of the possibility of a coagulopathy should be considered. In adolescents, heavy menstrual bleeding may be the first indication of a congenital bleeding tendency [36–38]. To evaluate this possibility, a complete blood count (CBC) with platelets, prothrombin time, and partial thromboplastin time are reasonable. Fibrinogen or thrombin time is optional. Data supports the observation that bleeding time is neither sensitive nor specific and is not indicated [39]. Depending on the outcomes of the initial tests, more specific tests for von Willebrand disease or other coagulopathies may be indicated (von Willebrand-ristocetin cofactor activity, von Willebrand factor antigen, and factor VIII).

Ultrasonographic imaging of the uterine cavity, wall, and environment may be helpful when secondary causes of heavy menstrual bleeding are being evaluated, such as a palpable abnormality during physical examination or initial treatment

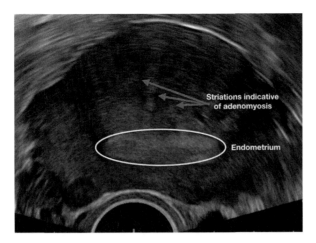

Fig. 8.6 Transvaginal ultrasonography of the uterus, showing the endometrium as a hyperechoic (brighter) area in the middle, with linear striations extending upward from it. This is a specific sign of adenomyosis

failure. For example, studies have demonstrated that the amount of menstrual bleeding is correlated with the number of ultrasonographic markers for adenomyosis [40]. Magnetic resonance imaging (MRI) should not be a primary imaging modality for heavy menstrual bleeding (Fig. 8.6).

Transabdominal ultrasonographic techniques may be adequate for selected or virginal patients. Transvaginal ultrasonography provides higher resolution (due to the higher frequency used by these transducers), but the field of view is shorter. This approach is best for the evaluation of adenomyosis or the endometrial cavity [41], and some have advocated that it be used in all patients with heavy menstrual bleeding [42], but that has yet to gain acceptance due to availability and cost. The addition of saline intracavitary infusion can improve the diagnostic accuracy for endometrial hyperplasia or polyps (Fig. 8.7).

The role of endometrial biopsy is generally limited to those patients where the possibility of endometrial hyperplasia or carcinoma is being considered, such as those over the age of 45. Some studies suggest that roughly 85% of endometrial biopsies obtained from women with a history of heavy menstrual bleeding will be normal [43]. Hysteroscopy allows direct viewing of endometrial cavity and the ability to take directed biopsies. Once again, this should be limited to patients where specific diagnoses are being considered, or initial therapies have failed, and not as an initial screening procedure.

Key Points
- The diagnosis of primary dysmenorrhea can generally be established by careful history.
- In young women with painful, but regular periods, a pelvic examination is not always necessary prior to starting treatment.

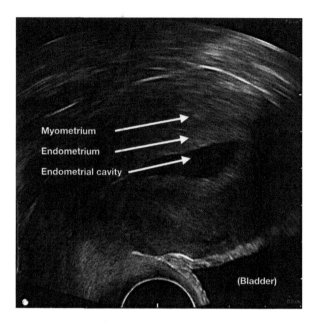

Fig. 8.7 Sonohysterography of the uterus of a 41-year-old woman. Sterile saline instilled into the cavity of the uterus is anechoic (dark), surrounded by the normal endometrium, seen as a hyperechoic (brighter) band around the cavity. This technique is particularly well suited for the diagnosis of endometrial and intracavitary lesions

- Because of the prevalence of pathologic causes for heavy menstrual bleeding, physical and laboratory evaluations, and imaging, play a bigger role in establishing the diagnosis.
- If intracavitary pathologies are likely in cases of heavy menstrual bleeding, saline infusion ultrasonography is the preferred imaging modality.
- Endometrial sampling should not be used as a screening tool for women with heavy menstrual bleeding.

References

1. Golding JM, Wilsnack SC, Learman LA. Prevalence of sexual assault history among women with common gynecologic symptoms. Am J Obstet Gynecol. 1998;179(4):1013–9.
2. Harada T, Momoeda M. Factors associated with increased pain in primary dysmenorrhea: analysis using a multivariate ordered logistic regression model. Fertil Steril. 2016;106(7):1807–14.
3. Hillen TIJ, Grbavac SL, Johnston PJ, Straton JAY, Keogh JMF. Primary dysmenorrhea in young western Australian women: prevalence, impact and knowledge of treatment. J Adolesc Health. 1999;25:40–5.
4. Balbi C, Musone R, Menditto A, et al. Influence of menstrual factors and dietary habits on menstrual pain in adolescence age. Eur J Obstet Gynecol Reprod Biol. 2000;91:143–8.

5. Burnett MA, Antao V, Black A, et al. Prevalence of primary dysmenorrhea in Canada. J Obstet Gynaecol Can. 2005;27(8):765–70.
6. Juang CM, Yen MS, Twu NF, Horng HC, Yu HC, Chen CY. Impact of pregnancy on primary dysmenorrhea. Int J Gynaecol Obstet. 2006;92(3):221–7.
7. Harlow BL, Missmer SA, Cramer DW, Barbieri RL. Does tubal sterilization influence the subsequent risk of menorrhagia or dysmenorrhea? Fertil Steril. 2002;77:754–60.
8. Sahin S, Ozdemir K, Unsal A, Arslan R. Review of frequency of dysmenorrhea and some associated factors and evaluation of the relationship between dysmenorrhea and sleep quality in university students. Gynecol Obstet Investig. 2014;78(3):179–85.
9. Johnson J. Level of knowledge among adolescent girls regarding effective treatment for dysmenorrhea. J Adolesc Health Care. 1988;9(5):398–402.
10. Campbell MA, McGrath PJ. Use of medication by adolescents for the management of menstrual discomfort. Arch Pediatr Adolesc Med. 1997;151(9):905–13.
11. O'Connell K, Davis AR, Westhoff C. Self-treatment patterns among adolescent girls with dysmenorrhea. J Pediatr Adolesc Gynecol. 2006;19:285–9.
12. Eskenazi B, Warner M, Bonsignore L, Olive D, Samuels S, Vercellini P. Validation study of nonsurgical diagnosis of endometriosis. Fertil Steril. 2001;76(5):929–35.
13. Fall M, Baranowski AP, Fowler CJ, et al. European Association of Urology. EAU guidelines on chronic pelvic pain. Eur Urol. 2004;46(6):681–9.
14. Kim J, Lee H, Kim H, Kim JY, Kim KH. Differences in the tongue features of primary dysmenorrhea patients and controls over a normal menstrual cycle. Evid Based Complement Alternat Med. 2017;2017:6435702.
15. Jeon SH, Kim KK, Lee IS, et al. Pulse wave variation during the menstrual cycle in women with menstrual pain. Biomed Res Int. 2016;2016:1083208.
16. American Institute of Ultrasound in Medicine. AIUM practice guideline for the performance of pelvic ultrasound examinations. J Ultrasound Med. 2010;29(1):166–72.
17. Hudelist G, English J, Thomas AE, Tinelli A, Singer CF, Keckstein J. Diagnostic accuracy of transvaginal ultrasound for non-invasive diagnosis of bowel endometriosis: systematic review and meta-analysis. Ultrasound Obstet Gynecol. 2011;37(3):257–63.
18. Saccardi C, Cosmi E, Borghero A, Tregneghi A, Dessole S, Litta P. Comparison between transvaginal sonography, saline contrast sonovaginography and magnetic resonance imaging in the diagnosis of posterior deep infiltrating endometriosis. Ultrasound Obstet Gynecol. 2012;40(4):464–9.
19. Hallberg L, Hogdahl AM, Nilsson L, Rybo G. Menstrual blood loss—a population study. Variation at different ages and attempts to define normality. Acta Obstet Gynecol Scand. 1966;45:320–51.
20. Hallberg L, Hogdahl AM, Nilsson L, et al. Menstrual blood loss and iron deficiency. Acta Med Scand. 1966;180:639–50.
21. Warner PE, Critchley HO, Lumsden MA, Campbell-Brown M, Douglas A, Murray GD. Menorrhagia II: is the 80-mL blood loss criterion useful in management of complaint of menorrhagia? Am J Obstet Gynecol. 2004;190:1224–9.
22. Cooper N, Barton P, Breijer M, et al. Cost-effectiveness of diagnostic strategies for the management of abnormal uterine bleeding (heavy menstrual bleeding and post-menopausal bleeding): a decision analysis. Health Technol Assess. 2014;18(24):1–201.
23. Chimbira TH, Anderson AB, Turnbull A. Relation between measured menstrual blood loss and patient's subjective assessment of loss, duration of bleeding, number of sanitary towels used, uterine weight and endometrial surface area. Br J Obstet Gynaecol. 1908;87(7):603–9.
24. Fraser IS, McCarron G, Markham R. A preliminary study of factors influencing perception of menstrual blood loss volume. Am J Obstet Gynecol. 1984;149(7):788–93.
25. Wyatt KM, Dimmock PW, Walker TJ, O'Brien PM. Determination of total menstrual blood loss. Fertil Steril. 2001;76:125–31.
26. Warner PE, Critchley HO, Lumsden MA, Campbell-Brown M, Douglas A, Murray GD, Menorrhagia I. Measured blood loss, clinical features, and outcome in women with heavy periods: a survey with follow-up data. Am J Obstet Gynecol. 2004;190:1216–23.

27. Schumacher U, Schumacher J, Mellinger U, Gerlinger C, Wienke A, Endrikat A. Estimation of menstrual blood loss volume based on menstrual diary and laboratory data. BMC Womens Health. 2012;12:24–31.
28. Rankin GLS, Veal N, Huntsman RG, Liddell J. Measurement with 51 Cr of red-cell loss in menorrhagia. Lancet. 1962;1(7229):567–9.
29. Higham JM, O'Brien PM, Shaw RW. Assessment of menstrual blood loss using a pictorial chart. Br J Obstet Gynaecol. 1908;97(8):734–9.
30. Janssen CA, Scholten PC, Heintz AP. A simple visual assessment technique to discriminate between menorrhagia and normal menstrual blood loss. Obstet Gynecol. 1995;85(6):977–82.
31. Zakherah MS, Sayed GH, El-Nashar SA, Shaaban MM. Pictorial blood loss assessment chart in the evaluation of heavy menstrual bleeding: diagnostic accuracy compared with alkaline hematin. Gynecol Obstet Investig. 2011;71(4):281–4.
32. Reid PC, Coker A, Coltart R. Assessment of menstrual blood loss using a pictorial chart: a validation study. BJOG. 2000;107:320–2.
33. Philipp CS, Faiz A, Dowling NF, et al. Development of a screening tool for identifying women with menorrhagia for hemostatic evaluation. Am J Obstet Gynecol. 2008;198:163.e1–8.
34. Milman N, Clausen J, Byg KE. Iron status in 268 Danish women aged 18-30 years: influence of menstruation, contraceptive method, and iron supplementation. Ann Hematol. 1998;77:13–9.
35. Working Party for Guidelines for the Management of Heavy Menstrual Bleeding. An evidence-based guideline for the management of heavy menstrual bleeding. New Zealand Med J. 1999;112:174–7.
36. Minjarez DA, Bradshaw KD. Abnormal uterine bleeding in adolescents. Obstet Gynecol Clin N Am. 2000;27:63–78.
37. Slap GB. Menstrual disorders in adolescence. Best Pract Res Clin Obstet Gynaecol. 2003;17:75–92.
38. Shankar M, Lee CA, Sabin CA, Economides DL, Kadir RA. Von Willebrand disease in women with menorrhagia: a systematic review. BJOG. 2004;111:734.
39. National Heart, Lung, and Blood Institute. The diagnosis, evaluation, and management of von Willebrand Disease. NIH Publication No. 08-5832. Bethesda, MD: NHLBI; 2007. Available at: http://www.nhlbi.nih.gov/guidelines/vwd/vwd.pdf. Accessed 11 July 2017
40. Naftalin J, Hoo W, Pateman K, Mavrelos D, Foo X, Jurkovic DI. Adenomyosis associated with menorrhagia? Hum Reprod. 2014;29(3):473–9.
41. Vercellini P, Cortesi I, Oldani S, Moschetta M, De Giorgi O, Crosignani PG. The role of trans-vaginal ultrasonography and outpatient diagnostic hysteroscopy in the evaluation of patients with menorrhagia. Hum Reprod. 1997;12(8):1768–71.
42. Wood C, Hurley VA, Leoni M. The value of vaginal ultrasound in the management of menorrhagia. Aust N Z J Obstet Gynaecol. 1993;33(2):198–200.
43. Ash SJ, Farrell SA, Flowerdew G. Endometrial biopsy in DUB. J Reprod Med. 1996;41(12):892–6.

Additional Resources

General overviews of the diagnosis of dysmenorrhea can be found at:
Allen LM, Lam AC. Premenstrual syndrome and dysmenorrhea in adolescents. Adolesc Med State Art Rev. 2012;23(1):139–63.
American College of Obstetricians and Gynecologists. Diagnosis of abnormal uterine bleeding in reproductive-aged women. Practice Bulletin No. 128. Obstet Gynecol. 2012;120:197–206.
American College of Obstetricians and Gynecologists. Hysteroscopy. Technology Assessment No. 7. Obstet Gynecol. 2011;117:1486–91.
American Institute of Ultrasound in Medicine. AIUM practice guideline for the performance of pelvic ultrasound examinations. J Ultrasound Med. 2010;29(1):166–72.

Dawood MY. Dysmenorrhea. J Reprod Med. 1985;30(3):154–67.

Dawood MY. Primary dysmenorrhea: advances in pathogenesis and management. Obstet Gynecol. 2006;108(2):428–41.

French L. Dysmenorrhea in adolescents: diagnosis and treatment. Paediatr Drugs. 2008;10(1):1–7.

Harel Z. Dysmenorrhea in adolescents. Ann N Y Acad Sci. 2008;1135:185–95.

Lefebvre G, Pinsonneault O, Antao V, et al. Primary dysmenorrhea consensus guideline. J Obstet Gynaecol Can. 2005;27(12):1117–46.

Proctor M, Farquhar C. Diagnosis and management of dysmenorrhoea. BMJ. 2006;332(7550):1134–8.

Schroeder B, Sanfilippo JS. Dysmenorrhea and pelvic pain in adolescents. Pediatr Clin N Am. 1999;46(3):555–71.

Smith RP. Netter's obstetrics & gynecology. 3rd ed. Philadelphia: Elsevier; 2017. p. 71–3.

Ylikorkala O, Dawood MY. New concepts in dysmenorrhea. Am J Obstet Gynecol. 1978;130(7):833–47.

Chapter 9
Management Strategies for Primary Dysmenorrhea

9.1 Topic Overview

In 1910, Dr. P. Brooke Bland wrote, "Dysmenorrhea should never be regarded as a morbid process, but should always be looked upon as a manifestation of some systemic or local pelvic condition. It is unfortunate that many women are operated upon for dysmenorrhea without the cause first being determined" [1]. In the past, therapies used to treat dysmenorrhea have ranged from the plausible and somewhat effective, to the outlandish and useless. Everything from cauterizing the middle turbinate of the nose [2], exercise programs [3], and presacral sympathectomy [4, 5] to uterine relaxing factor [6], vasodilators [7, 8], tranquilizers [9], and hormones [10, 11] have been recommended to relieve dysmenorrhea. The use of electric current has even been advocated [12], employing an insulated chair, an intravaginal electrode, and a spark gap high-voltage generator. This treatment was to be administered for 20 min daily over a 4-week period. The treatment was reported to have had good effects, possibly do to a low return rate of patients treated in this way (Fig. 9.1).

Today, the symptoms of primary dysmenorrhea may be effectively prevented with the use of nonsteroidal anti-inflammatory agents or hormonal manipulations of the endometrium. Newer treatments of the conditions that secondarily cause menstrual pain, such as uterine leiomyomata or endometriosis, also have more effective, less invasive, or intrusive treatments to provide relief. Because the treatments of secondary dysmenorrhea are varied and determined by the causative process, they are beyond the scope of this text. General resources for many of those processes are listed under additional resources at the end of this chapter.

© Springer International Publishing AG 2018
R.P. Smith, *Dysmenorrhea and Menorrhagia*,
https://doi.org/10.1007/978-3-319-71964-1_9

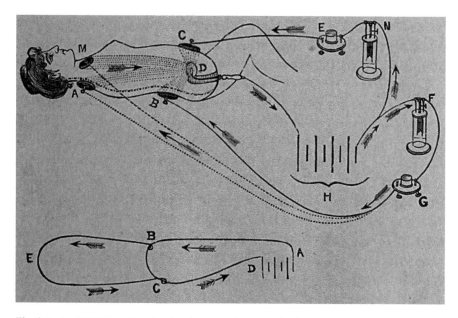

Fig. 9.1 An 1888 illustration for the electrode placement for intrauterine galvanism showing a battery and a "water rheostat" for adjusting the current [13]. (H. battery, N. water rheostat, E. milliamperemeter, D. intrauterine pole (active), C. abdominal pole (dispersing) of the primary circuit, K. point where circuit branches, F. water rheostat, G. milliamperemeter; B and A. lumbar and spinal pole can be placed over cervical sympathetic as at M. D. intrauterine pole. I. point of return to primary circuit of the derived current)

9.2 Pharmacologic Therapies

It would seem logical that if prostaglandin synthesis can be reduced, menstrual pain could be prevented or lessened. In 1967, Pickles showed that prostaglandin levels were less during anovulatory cycles [14]. This prompted the use of oral contraceptives to suppress ovulation and relieve menstrual pain [10, 11]. While this approach is usually successful, not all patients want to, or can, take oral contraceptives. The recognition of the anti-prostaglandin effects of the nonsteroidal anti-inflammatory drugs (NSAIDs), and the use of these effective agents, has resulted in a much more direct way of altering the pathophysiology of primary dysmenorrhea.

For women with primary dysmenorrhea, the documented efficacy of NSAIDs and hormonal therapies has meant that the promise of pain prevention, not pain relief, has become a reality. Through both subjective and objective means, these interventions have documented impact on the underlying pathophysiology of primary dysmenorrhea [15–18].

9.2.1 Nonsteroidal Anti-inflammatory Agents

Treatment of primary dysmenorrhea with NSAIDs has become the accepted initial management [19, 20]. The choice of agents should be driven by factors such as cost, duration of action, presence, and type of side effects associated with the agent, and documented efficacy. Attempts to summarize published studies have been unable to provide clear guidance based upon efficacy alone [19, 21, 22]. It should be borne in mind that drugs from a given class of agents will generally have similar performance and characteristics as others in the same family (see Chap. 7). Patients with aspirin-sensitive asthma, ulcers, or inflammatory bowel disease should not use these drugs. Prolonged use of NSAIDs is associated with an increased risk of renal damage, but the short exposure required to treat dysmenorrhea makes this unlikely.

Some drugs that have the ability to inhibit prostaglandin synthesis have had little clinical usefulness: some have weak anti-prostaglandin activity, require metabolic transformation to become active, or have side effects which limit their usefulness. These drugs (such as aspirin, phenacetin, phenylbutazone, paracetamol, or indomethacin) can be used to treat dysmenorrhea but have generally been superseded by more effective agents.

Older members of the enolic acid NSAIDs, such as piroxicam or meloxicam, are limited to veterinary applications or for limited use in chronic inflammatory conditions and are not appropriate for dysmenorrhea therapy. The coxib family of predominantly cyclooxygenase-2 inhibitors enjoyed some use in treating dysmenorrhea following their introduction, until the recognition of significant cardiovascular side effects. Most of these drugs have been withdrawn from the US market. Those that remain do not have an FDA indication for the treatment of dysmenorrhea (Fig. 9.2).

It is the carboxylates that most physicians are familiar with and have the most day-to-day use for pain relief and dysmenorrhea. The most recognized agent in this group, aspirin, has a very low potency for reducing prostaglandin synthesis in the uterus and, hence, has had little clinical utility in the treatment of moderate or severe dysmenorrhea. Increased potency is seen in the acetic acid group. While sulindac

---

WARNING: RISK OF SERIOUS CARDIOVASCULAR AND GASTROINTERSTINAL EVENTS
See full prescribing information for complete boxed warning.

- Nonsteroidal anti-inflammatory drugs (NSAIDs) cause an increased risk of serious cardiovascular thrombotic events, including myocardial infarction and stroke, which can be fatal. This risk may occur early in the treatment and may increase with duration of use.
- CELEBREX is contraindicated in the setting of coronary artery bypass graft (CABG) surgery.
- NSAIDs cause an increased risk of serious gastrointestinal (GI) adverse events including bleeding, ulceration, and perforation of the stomach or intestines, which can be fatal. These events can occur at any time during use and without warning symptoms. Elderly patients and patients with a prior history of peptic ulcer disease and/ or GI bleeding are at greater risk for serious GI events.

Fig. 9.2 The current "black box warning" required by the FDA to accompany the prescribing information for celecoxib (Celebrex)

must undergo reduction to a sulfide form before becoming active, most of the drugs in this group are directly effective as anti-inflammatory and analgesic agents. In several studies, indomethacin has shown usefulness in treating dysmenorrhea [23–26], but a moderate incidence of side effects has limited the use of this, and most other drugs in this class, for treating dysmenorrhea.

The most commonly used drugs for dysmenorrhea come from the two remaining carboxylate groups: propionic acid derivatives (arylalkanoic acids) and anthranilic acids (fenamates). Ibuprofen, ketoprofen, meclofenamate, mefenamic acid, and naproxen are the NSAIDs specifically approved by the US Food and Drug Administration (FDA) for treatment of dysmenorrhea, though other agents have been used and reported (Table 9.1).

The arylalkanoic acids, ibuprofen and naproxen, are widely available without prescription in the United States, while ketoprofen has limited use even by prescription. While there are no therapeutic differences between the over-the-counter (OTC) and prescription formulations of these drugs, for effective dysmenorrhea therapy, the patient must take multiple doses of the OTC formulations and often exceed the

Table 9.1 Approved dysmenorrhea therapies (U.S.)

Drug	Typical trade name	Initial dosage	Continuing dosage	Comments
Ibuprofen	Motrin, Advil, NeoProfen, Brufen, and others	400–800 mg	400 mg q4h	Typical over-the-counter dose is 200 mg per caplet, with a warning not to exceed six caplets in 24 h, requiring the patient to use multiple caplets and ignore this warning
Ketoprofen	Orudis KT, Actron	75 mg	75 mg t.i.d.	Ketoprofen was available over-the-counter in the United States, but this form has been discontinued. Used primarily for topical and veterinary applications
Naproxen/ naproxen sodium	Aleve, Naprosyn, Anaprox, and others	500 mg/550 mg	250 mg q6–8h/275 mg q6–8h	Naproxen may have antiviral activity against influenza
Meclofenamate sodium	Meclomen	100 mg	50–100 mg q6h	Rapid onset of action in humans results in an increased rate of gastrointestinal side effects
Mefenamic acid	Ponstel, Ponstan, Ponalar	500 mg	250 mg q4–6h	Data suggests that mefenamic acid may be able to bind to the PGE receptor, blocking the action of prostaglandins after their formation

labeled recommendations. For patients with milder symptoms, these over-the-counter options are good choices. For more severe symptoms, the prescription strengths of these agents should be choosen.

The anthranilic acid derivatives, meclofenamate sodium and mefenamic acid, are more expensive and less widely used NSIADs for dysmenorrhea, but a dual mode of action has been demonstrated for fenamates, which reduce prostaglandin synthesis and inhibit binding of PGE_2 to its receptor [27]. In vitro studies have shown that meclofenamate can inhibit the activity of 5-lipoxygenase, while members of the propionic acid group have little or no inhibitory ability [28–30]. The clinical significance of this inhibition of leukotrienes is not known. Objective measures of the impact of mefenamic acid on uterine activity do show that changes in uterine activity can be seen as quickly as 15 min after dosing [16, 18]. This rapid effect requires speedy absorption from the stomach, resulting in higher rates of gastrointestinal side effects (Fig. 9.3).

The overall success of NSAIDs in treating primary dysmenorrhea has been well documented. Owen [26] presented data from 51 reports and attempted to analyze the diverse methods, designs, and outcomes in the studies reported to that time. She found an 87% "excellent" pain relief for the fenamates versus 56%, 68%, and 56% for ibuprofen, indomethacin, and naproxen, respectively. Differences in study design, dependent variables, inclusion and exclusion criteria, and the very nature of subjective pain studies make it inevitable that no clear guidance regarding the first choice for agents has emerged.

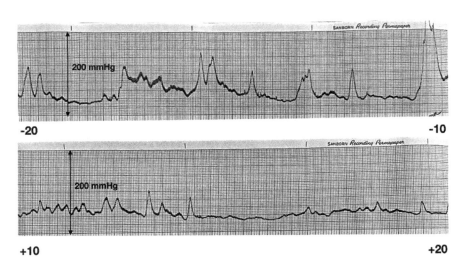

Fig. 9.3 A portion of intrauterine pressure recordings covering a roughly 10-min period before blinded treatment with meclofenamate sodium (−20 to −10 min, above) and following ingestion of the drug (+10 to +20 min, below). The full-scale pressure recording is 200 mmHg in each case. Even over the 10-min segment shown, the evolution of the uterine activity improvement is apparent

Few direct comparisons of one drug to another have been carried out. While most of these have shown superiority of the active drug over placebo and occasionally shown trends favoring one drug or another, no study has had sufficient statistical power to separate the efficacies of the active agents tested [19]. It is safe to say, however, that failure of these agents to accomplish at least some improvement in symptoms should prompt a reevaluation of the diagnosis [31].

9.2.2 Hormonal Therapies

Early studies established that the use of combination oral contraceptives (COCs) reduced menstrual prostaglandins by limiting endometrial development [32]. Clinical experience and multiple studies [33, 34] support combination hormonal contraceptives as reasonable primary or secondary therapies for women who are not currently trying to conceive. As with the NSAIDs, no clear-cut evidence exists to prefer one formulation over another. A review of randomized trials comparing the contraceptive vaginal ring with COCs concluded that both had a similar improvement in dysmenorrhea symptoms [35] (Fig. 9.4).

Combination contraceptives can be administered in monthly cycles, in extended cycles, or continuously. The use of long-cycle or flexible regimen oral contraceptives for dysmenorrhea is attractive for the treatment of both heavy menstrual bleeding and pain. Studies have demonstrated good response [37]. Similarly, even ultra-low-dose oral contraceptives can be effective [36], reducing hormone load in those where this might be a consideration. The major disadvantage to the use of long- or extended-cycle therapy is that many women develop breakthrough spotting or bleeding, limiting acceptance and continuation. Accordingly, counseling women

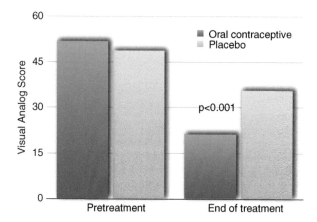

Fig. 9.4 In a study of 158 women with dysmenorrhea treated with oral contraceptives (105 women) and placebo (53 women), the use of a combination oral contraceptive agent resulted in a statistically significant reduction in menstrual pain [36]

regarding this common side effect will improve patient satisfaction and continuation of this approach to reducing dysmenorrhea.

Depot medroxyprogesterone acetate, implantable contraceptive capsules, and the levonorgestrel-releasing intrauterine contraceptive device (LNG-IUD) represent alternatives to combination hormonal contraceptives. Reviews of published studies suggest that the LNG-IUD is equal or superior to systemic progestins or oral contraceptives for the treatment of dysmenorrhea [38] and appears to be particularly well suited to adolescents [39]. In a large 3-year trial assessing the safety and efficacy of the single-rod etonogestrel-releasing implantable contraceptive, over 75% of participants who reported primary dysmenorrhea at baseline had improvement in their symptoms [40]. In another trial, the single-rod contraceptive implant was associated with a 68% reduction of dysmenorrhea [41].

The use of cyclic oral progesterone to treat dysmenorrhea has been reported in the older literature. In one trial of 150 student nurses treated with either the progestin dydrogesterone or placebo, 81% of those taking the placebo had to resort to using a rescue analgesic, while only 2% of the progesterone group needed the analgesic [42]. There were 12 episodes of breakthrough bleeding among four patients in the dydrogesterone group (4% of patients). Just as oral progesterone-only contraceptive methods have a limited, but useful, place in contraceptive management, breakthrough bleeding and uncertain contraceptive efficacy have limited oral progesterone therapy for dysmenorrhea (Fig. 9.5).

9.2.3 Other Pharmacologic Therapies

Nitric oxide, nitroglycerin, and calcium channel blockers all have tocolytic effects, making them logical options, and have been investigated as potential therapies of dysmenorrhea. Side effects and the availability of other agents have meant that there is no current role for these drugs.

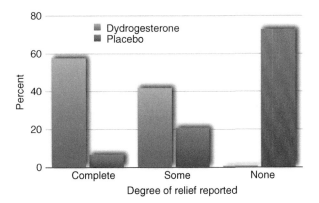

Fig. 9.5 The degree of symptom relief obtained by 150 dysmenorrheic student nurses treated in a double-blind, placebo-controlled study of dydrogesterone (10 mg, twice daily) administered from days 5 to 20 of the menstrual cycle [42]. The study covered 12 cycles, 6 on each treatment, for each subject

Table 9.2 Therapeutic approaches to primary dysmenorrhea

Strategy	Method	Advantages	Disadvantages
Prostaglandin suppression	Non-steroidal anti-inflammatory drugs	Widely available, proven effective in reducing uterine activity and subjective pain, some agents available without prescription	Risk of gastrointestinal upset, prescription required for optimal dosing or some agents
Ovulation suppression	Hormonal manipulation	Provides contraception, regular bleeding, reduced flow	Prolonged medication exposure for 2–4 days of relief, prescription required
Endometrial suppression	Topical hormone treatment (IUD)	Provides contraception, reduced flow, possibly absent menses	Expense, more invasive (placement and removal), possibility of random bleeding
Topical heat	Heat patch	Non-prescription, no systemic side effects, proven effectiveness, effective for 8–10 h, discrete	Expense, effectiveness reduced if heat patch is deprived of oxygen
Transcutaneous electrical nerve stimulation (TENS)	TENS unit	Effective, patient controlled, non-pharmacologic	Expense, availability, equipment required
Lifestyle modification	Diet, exercise	Overall health benefits, inexpensive	Limited data on efficacy
Complementary and alternative medicine	Acupuncture, traditional herbal medications	Desirability by some patients, some data to support benefits	Access, portability, and limited data

By inhibiting phosphodiesterase, myometrial blood flow can be enhanced, causing a reduction in primary dysmenorrhea. A small randomized, double-blind trial of the efficacy of a vaginal preparation of sildenafil citrate (100 mg single dose) was reported to improve primary dysmenorrhea compared to placebo [43]. Unfortunately, the study was not able to meet its recruitment goals to establish statistical power, so the findings are not conclusive (Table 9.2).

9.3 Non-pharmacologic Treatments

Many patients use non-pharmacologic methods to ameliorate their dysmenorrhea symptoms, from 25% to up to 96% of patients in some studies [44, 45]. Some of the methods are traditional, some idiosyncratic, and some unconventional. They range from the innocuous to more invasive. Response rates are often variable, and only a few have been well studied. When patients seek advice surrounding these interventions, it is reasonable to recommend those with efficacy as adjuncts or supplements to other modalities. Unfortunately, the majority of users of these approaches use them in combinations and do not seek professional guidance [46] (Fig. 9.6).

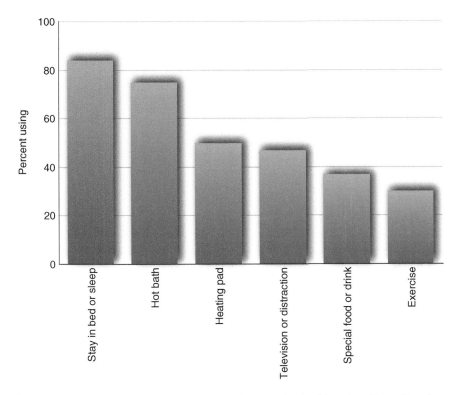

Fig. 9.6 Non-pharmacologic remedies used for dysmenorrhea by 76 study subjects. Data from O'Connell et al. [46]

9.3.1 Heat

The use of heat to treat dysmenorrhea has a historical record of success and storied folklore but low levels of practical use. Despite acknowledged utility, for a long time, heat therapy lacked any rigorous or systematic evaluation in the scientific literature, with only sporadic case reports [47]. The practicalities of rapidly cooling hot-water bottles, electrical cords, and the risk of burns from heating pads have limited the utility of this option. The development of small, wearable devices capable of supplying a continuous low level of heat now makes this a viable option. Published studies have demonstrated that continuous low-level heat was similar or superior to oral ibuprofen [48] or acetaminophen [49]. Heat therapy can be combined with other treatments, such as transcutaneous electrical nerve stimulation (TENS), with good effect [50] (Fig. 9.7).

Unlike NSAIDs, which are more effective for primary dysmenorrhea and which may cause gastrointestinal upset, heat therapy should be equally effective in many cases of secondary dysmenorrhea. Topical heat therapy can be used safely in those patients with known or suspected gastrointestinal disorders, where NSAIDs might be contraindicated.

Fig. 9.7 This French pewter hot-water bottle (c. 1751–1810 CE) is engraved with birds and plants and has a curved shape to fit close against the body. (Image: Wellcome Library, London. Wellcome Images)

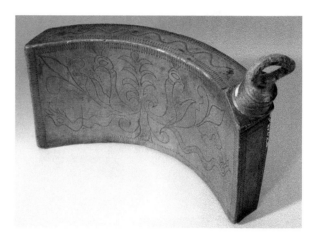

9.3.2 Transcutaneous Electrical Nerve Stimulation

Transcutaneous electrical nerve stimulation uses pulsed electrical current to alter the perception of pain. A typical battery-operated TENS unit is able to modulate pulse width, frequency, and intensity through user controls. Generally, the current is high frequency (>50 Hz) with an intensity below that required to stimulate muscle contraction.

Transcutaneous electrical nerve stimulation is thought to raise the threshold for pain signals by sending afferent impulses through the large-diameter sensory fibers of the nerve root, resulting in lower perception of painful uterine signals and stimulating the release of endorphins from the peripheral nerves and the spinal cord [51–53]. Intrauterine pressure studies indicate that TENS therapy has no significant effect on uterine contractile activity [53, 54], underscoring a direct effect on the perception of pain.

A meta-analysis found that high-frequency TENS was more effective than placebo TENS for relief of dysmenorrhea [55], and many single studies report rapid onset of relief [56]. Therefore, TENS appears to be a useful alternative for women who cannot, or prefer not to, take NSAIDs or oral contraceptive. If the degree of pain relief obtained with TENS therapy alone is incomplete [57], some women may be able to lower their analgesic dose with combined therapy [58] or with heat combined with TENS [50, 59] (Fig. 9.8).

9.4 Lifestyle Modification

Lifestyle, dietary, wellness, and complementary medical treatments have all been advocated for the treatment of dysmenorrhea [60]. Though generally less effective and less well studied than pharmaceutical interventions, heat, or TENS, their cost

Fig. 9.8 One of several reported placement patterns of TENS electrodes for the treatment of dysmenorrhea symptoms using a dual-channel unit [54]. For women with predominantly back symptoms, placement of the electrodes over the low back may be more effective

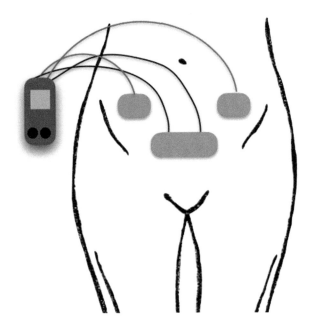

and other benefits recommend that they be considered for selected patients and as adjuncts in others.

9.4.1 Dietary Interventions

A variety of dietary and vitamin therapies may reduce the severity of menstrual pain, but data are limited to a few small studies. These include low-fat vegetarian diets; vitamins E, B_1, B_6, and D; fish oil supplements; and Japanese herbal combinations. Three small, randomized trials found that magnesium was more effective than placebo for relief of dysmenorrhea and was well tolerated [61], but the small size of the trials, high dropout rates, and varying designs precluded a definite recommendation for use of magnesium.

Four randomized trials have compared the therapeutic efficacy of ginger with a placebo during the first 3–4 days of the menstrual cycle. Collectively, these studies provide suggestive evidence for the effectiveness of 750–2000 mg ginger powder for primary dysmenorrhea [62]. However, a recent review concluded that, while efficacy has been documented, the results need to be interpreted with caution because of the small number of studies, poor methodological quality, and high heterogeneity across trials [63] (Fig. 9.9).

An uncontrolled study of vitamin E supplementation reported improvement in symptoms, but methodologic concerns limit the applicability of the report [64]. The use of fish oil and calcium supplementation has been reported, but the results were

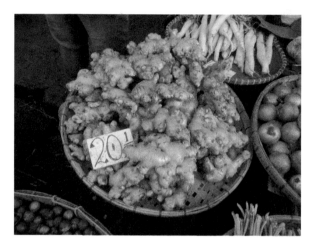

Fig. 9.9 Ginger root (*Zingiber officinale*), in fresh or powdered form, has been a traditional remedy in many cultures

unremarkable [65]. Overall, there is no high-quality evidence to support the effectiveness of any dietary supplement for dysmenorrhea, and evidence of safety is lacking [66]. Despite this, there is no reason not to recommend a healthy diet and lifestyle.

9.4.2 Exercise

The role of exercise to either improve or worsen menstrual pain is unclear. A systematic review on the use of exercise for relief included a single randomized trial [67] that documented improvements [68]. Most observational studies have reported decreased prevalence of dysmenorrhea and/or improved symptomatology with exercise [69]. However, the quality of this trial and these studies was low. One study has suggested that noncompetitive activities provide greater relief than when competition is an element [70]. Yoga [71, 72] and sexual activity may be helpful. Anecdotal experience suggests that menses-related discomfort is relieved by orgasm in some women [73] and is lower in those with more frequent intercourse [74], though attitudes and practices may affect the adoption of this finding [75, 76]. Overall, the variable nature of the exercise trials reported, and the difficulty in establishing benefit, has limited the ability to make informed recommendations [77, 78].

9.4.3 Complementary and Alternative Therapies

Fischer and colleagues have published a review of complementary and alternative medicine treatments for dysmenorrhea [79]. They found that herbal medicine, nutritional supplements, and massage are widely used, but a large number of these

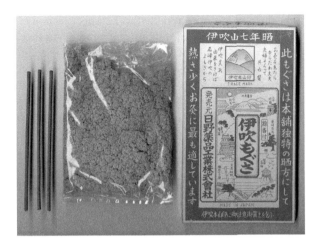

Fig. 9.10 Moxibustion is a traditional Chinese medicine therapy, which consists of burning dried mugwort (*moxa*) on particular points on the body—the abdomen in the case of menstrual cramps. Shown is a traditional moxibustion set from Japan where *mogusa* has been produced for centuries. A thick incense stick is used to light the *moxa* cones made from this material. (Image: Wellcome Library, London. Wellcome Images)

modalities are begun, often simultaneously, with little or no professional oversight.

Although acupuncture has been a traditional for treatment of dysmenorrhea, the studies reported have been of low quality and vary widely in design [80] with some showing statistical, but clinically insignificant, changes [81]. Accordingly, a 2016 meta-analysis of 42 trials on acupuncture or acupressure was unable to determine if acupuncture or acupressure was effective in treating primary dysmenorrhea [82]. Injections into acupuncture points have been reported to be of value in a double-blind double-dummy trial [83].

A pragmatic trial of moxibustion demonstrated effectiveness, but not the efficacy, for menstrual pain. It could not rule out the confounding effect of psychological factors, because of a lack of blinding or sham controls [84]. A randomized trial was more convincing [85], but the role for this approach to treatment still seems limited (Fig. 9.10).

Chinese and Japanese herbal medicines have also enjoyed a long history of use for dysmenorrhea, but data surrounding their efficacy has been variable [61]. A systematic review of 39 randomized trials found this approach to be promising compared to other therapies, but no firm conclusions could be made due to poor methodologic quality of the trials [86]. Despite this lack of consensus, these agents are still widely used [87].

The use of spinal manipulation has been reported [88] and explored in a meta-analysis that showed the technique was no more effective than sham manipulation for the treatment of primary dysmenorrhea [89].

Low-level light therapy has been reported to be effective in a small trial [90], though the results were only statistically significant when controlled for age, which has been shown to have its own effect on dysmenorrhea. The addition of rose oil aromatherapy to diclofenac has been reported, but the changes noted were limited [91]. Lastly, the use of hypnosis has been reported to be comparable to medical management at 3 months [92], but the lack of controls, the use of an only three-point rating scale, and other methodologic issues limit the conclusions that can be reached.

9.5   Surgical Treatment

Surgical treatments have little role in the initial treatment of primary menstrual pain. For most patients, surgical therapy is restricted to the treatment of secondary dysmenorrhea causes or refractory cases where less invasive options have been exhausted. For this reason, the discussion of surgical options is reserved for Chap. 11—"Options for When Simple Managements Are Not Enough."

Key Points
- The most effective pharmacologic intervention with the lowest drug exposure remains the nonsteroidal anti-inflammatory agents (NSAIDs).
- For those wishing concomitant contraception, or who cannot use NSAIDs, combination oral contraceptives give good cycle control with reductions in both pain and menstrual flow volume.
- Long-cycle progesterone-based contraceptive will also provide improved menstrual experiences but with less reliable cycle control, often resulting in patient dissatisfaction or method change.
- Topical continuous low-level heat applied to the lower abdomen has been shown to have comparable efficacy to the NSAIDs for many patients, has no reported side effects, and can be combined with other modalities.
- Transcutaneous electrical nerve stimulation (TENS) can be effective in relieving menstrual pain through blocking the perception of pain, rather than altering prostaglandin production or uterine activity.
- For selected patients, complementary and alternative medical treatments may be useful.

References

1. Bland PB. Dysmenorrhea; its significance and treatment. J Med Soc NJ. 1910;6(12):591–4.
2. Mayer E. The intranasal treatment of dysmenorrhea. With a report of ninety-three cases. JAMA. 1914;62(1):6–8.
3. Miller NF, Berkman SJ. Dysmenorrhea. Amer. J Obstet Gynecol. 1953;65:505–16.
4. Cotte G. La sympathectomie hypogastrique: A-t-elle sa place dans latherapeutique gynecologique? Presse Med. 1925;33:98–102.

5. Black WT Jr. Use of presacral sympathectomy in the treatment of dysmenorrhea: a second look after twenty-five years. Am J Obstet Gynecol. 1964;89:16–22.
6. Hayden GE. Relief of primary dysmenorrhea. Obstet Gynecol. 1960;16:730–3.
7. Schuck F. Pain and pain relief in essential dysmenorrhea. Am J Obstet Gynecol. 1951;62(3):559–67.
8. Voulgaris DM. Dysmenorrhea. Treatment with Isoxsuprine. Obstet Gynecol. 1960;15:220–2.
9. Champlin WD, Corbit JP. Chlorpromazine and chlorpromazine combinations in the treatment of dysmenorrhea. Am J Obstet Gynecol. 1957;74(2):419–21.
10. Filler W. The treatment of dysmenorrhea. With special reference to the primary type. Med Clin North Am. 1951;35:861–70.
11. Menaker JS, Powers KD. Management of primary dysmenorrhea. Obstet Gynecol. 1962;20:66–71.
12. Torbett JW. The diagnosis and office treatment of some gynecologic cases. Texas State J Med. 1902;4(9):224–6.
13. Hulbert GT. Electricity vs. tait, or the use of electricity in inflammation as found in gynecology. St. Louis Courier of Medicine. 1888;20(3):193–217. (shown: Figures 1–2, p. 207)
14. Pickles VR. Prostaglandins in the human endometrium. Int J Fertil. 1967;12:335–8.
15. Smith RP, Powell JR. The objective evaluation of dysmenorrhea therapy. Am J Obstet Gynecol. 1980;137:314–9.
16. Smith RP, Powell JR. Intrauterine pressure changes during mefenamic acid treatment of primary spasmodic dysmenorrhea. Am J Obstet Gynecol. 1982;143:286–92.
17. Smith RP, Powell JR. Simultaneous objective and subjective evaluation of meclofenamate sodium in the treatment of primary dysmenorrhea. Am J Obstet Gynecol. 1987;157(3):611–6.
18. Smith RP. The dynamics of nonsteroidal anti-inflammatory therapy for primary dysmenorrhea. Obstet Gynecol. 1987;70(5):7858.
19. Marjoribanks J, Ayeleke RO, Farquhar C, Proctor M. Nonsteroidal anti-inflammatory drugs for dysmenorrhoea. Cochrane Database Syst Rev. 2015;(7):CD001751.
20. Zahradnik HP, Hanjalic-Beck A, Groth K. Nonsteroidal anti-inflammatory drugs and hormonal contraceptives for pain relief from dysmenorrhea: a review. Contraception. 2010;81(3):185–96.
21. Dawood MY. Nonsteroidal antiinflammatory drugs and reproduction. Am J Obstet Gynecol. 1993;169:1255–65.
22. Zhang WY, Po ALW. Efficacy of minor analgesics in primary dysmenorrhoea: a systematic review. Br J Obstet Gynaecol. 1998;105:780–9.
23. Lundström V. Treatment of primary dysmenorrhea with prostaglandin synthetase inhibitors—a promising therapeutic alternative. Acta Obstet Gynecol Scand. 1978;57(5):421–8.
24. Dingfelder JR. Primary dysmenorrhea treatment with prostaglandin inhibitors: a review. Am J Obstet Gynecol. 1981;140(8):874–9.
25. Gookin KS, Forman ES, Vecchio TJ, Wiser WL, Morrison JC. Comparative efficacy of ibuprofen, indomethacin, and placebo in the treatment of primary dysmenorrhea. South Med J. 1983;76(11):1361–2. 1367
26. Owen PR. Prostaglandin synthetase inhibitors in the treatment of primary dysmenorrhea. Am J Obstet Gynecol. 1984;148:96–103.
27. Rees MC, Cañete-Solér R, López Bernal A, Turnbull AC. Effect of fenamates on prostaglandin E receptor binding. Lancet. 1988;2(8610):541–2.
28. Casey FB, Appleby BJ, Buck DC. Selective inhibition of the lipoxygenase metabolic pathway of arachidonic acid by the SRA-A antagonist, FPL 55712. Prostaglandins. 1983;25:1–11.
29. Myers RF, Siegel MI. Differential effects of anti-inflammatory drugs on lipoxygenase and cyclooxygenase activities of neutrophils from a reverse passive Arthus reaction. Biochem Biophys Res Commun. 1983;112:586–94.
30. Boctor AM, Eickholt M, Pugsley TA. Meclofenamate sodium is an inhibitor of both the 5-Lipoxygenase and cyclooxygenase pathways of the arachidonic acid cascade *in vitro*. Prostaglandins Leukot Med. 1986;23:229–38.
31. Harel Z. Dysmenorrhea in adolescents and young adults: an update on pharmacological treatments and management strategies. Expert Opin Pharmacother. 2012;13(15):2157–70.

32. Chan WY, Dawood MY, Fuchs F. Prostaglandins in primary dysmenorrhea. Comparison of prophylactic and nonprophylactic treatment with ibuprofen and use of oral contraceptives. Am J Med. 1981;70(3):535–41.
33. Lindh I, Ellström AA, Milsom I. The effect of combined oral contraceptives and age on dysmenorrhoea: an epidemiological study. Hum Reprod. 2012;27(3):676–82.
34. Wong CL, Farquhar C, Roberts H, Proctor M. Oral contraceptive pill for primary dysmenorrhoea. Cochrane Database Syst Rev. 2009;(4):CD002120.
35. Roumen FJ. The contraceptive vaginal ring compared with the combined oral contraceptive pill: a comprehensive review of randomized controlled trials. Contraception. 2007;75:420–9.
36. Harada T, Momoeda M. Evaluation of an ultra-low-dose oral contraceptive for dysmenorrhea: a placebo-controlled, double-blind, randomized trial. Fertil Steril. 2016;106(7):1807–14.
37. Momoeda M, Kondo M, Elliesen J, Yasuda M, Yamamoto S, Harada T. Efficacy and safety of a flexible extended regimen of ethinylestradiol/drospirenone for the treatment of dysmenorrhea: a multicenter, randomized, open-label, active-controlled study. Int J Womens Health. 2017;9:295–305.
38. Imai A, Matsunami K, Takagi H, Ichigo S. Levonorgestrel-releasing intrauterine device used for dysmenorrhea: five-year literature review. Clin Exp Obstet Gynecol. 2014;41(5):495–8.
39. Gold MA, Johnson LM. Intrauterine devices and adolescents. Curr Opin Obstet Gynecol. 2008;20(5):464–9.
40. Croxatto HB. Clinical profile of Implanon: a single-rod etonogestrel contraceptive implant. Eur J Contracept Reprod Health Care. 2000;5(Suppl 2):21–8.
41. Walch K, Unfried G, Huber J, et al. Implanon versus medroxyprogesterone acetate: effects on pain scores in patients with symptomatic endometriosis—a pilot study. Contraception. 2009;79:29–34.
42. Aydar CK, Coleman BD. Treatment of primary dysmenorrhea: a double blind study. JAMA. 1965;192(11):161–3.
43. Dmitrovic R, Kunselman AR, Legro RS. Sildenafil citrate in the treatment of pain in primary dysmenorrhea: a randomized controlled trial. Hum Reprod. 2013;28:2958–65.
44. Aktaş D. Prevalence and factors affecting dysmenorrhea in female university students: effect on general comfort level. Pain Manag Nurs. 2015;16(4):534–43.
45. De Sanctis V, Soliman AT, Elsedfy H, Soliman NA, Soliman R, El Kholy M. Dysmenorrhea in adolescents and young adults: a review in different country. Acta Biomed. 2017;87(3):233–46.
46. O'Connell K, Davis AR, Westhoff C. Self-treatment patterns among adolescent girls with dysmenorrhea. J Pediatr Adolesc Gynecol. 2006;19:285–9.
47. Vance AR, Hayes SH, Spielholz NI. Microwave diathermy treatment for primary dysmenorrhea. Phys Ther. 1996;76:1003–8.
48. Akin MD, Weingand KW, Hengehold DA, Goodale MB, Hinkle RT, Smith RP. Use of continuous low-level topical heat in the treatment of dysmenorrhea. Obstet Gynecol. 2001;97:343–9.
49. Akin MD, Price W, Rodriguez G Jr, Erasala G, Hurley G, Smith RP. Continuous low-level topical heat wrap therapy compared to acetaminophen for primary dysmenorrhea. J Reprod Med. 2004;49:739–45.
50. Lee B, Hong SH, Kim K, et al. Efficacy of the device combining high-frequency transcutaneous electrical nerve stimulation and thermotherapy for relieving primary dysmenorrhea: a randomized, single-blind, placebo-controlled trial. Eur J Obstet Gynecol Reprod Biol. 2015;194:58–63.
51. Lundeberg T, Bondesson L, Lundström V. Relief of primary dysmenorrhea by transcutaneous electrical nerve stimulation. Acta Obstet Gynecol Scand. 1985;64(6):491–7.
52. Dawood MY. Primary dysmenorrhea: advances in pathogenesis and management. Obstet Gynecol. 2006;108:428.
53. Milsom I, Hedner N, Mannheimer CA. Comparative study of the effect of high-intensity transcutaneous nerve stimulation and oral naproxen on intrauterine pressure and menstrual pain in patients with primary dysmenorrhea. Am J Obstet Gynecol. 1994;170(1 Pt 1):123–9.
54. Smith RP, Heltzel J. Interrelation of analgesia and uterine activity in women with primary dysmenorrhea. A preliminary report. J Reprod Med. 1991;36:260–4.

55. Proctor ML, Smith CA, Farquhar CM, Stones RW. Transcutaneous electrical nerve stimulation and acupuncture for primary dysmenorrhoea (Cochrane review). Cochrane Database Syst Rev. 2002;(1):CD002123.
56. Wang SF, Lee JP, Hwa HL. Effect of transcutaneous electrical nerve stimulation on primary dysmenorrhea. Neuromodulation. 2009;12(4):302–9.
57. Kaplan B, Peled Y, Pardo J, et al. Transcutaneous electrical nerve stimulation (TENS) as a relief for dysmenorrhea. Clin Exp Obstet Gynecol. 1994;21(2):87–90.
58. Dawood MY, Ramos J. Transcutaneous electrical nerve stimulation (TENS) for the treatment of primary dysmenorrhea: a randomized crossover comparison with placebo TENS and ibuprofen. Obstet Gynecol. 1990;75(4):656–60.
59. Igwea SE, Tabansi-Ochuogu CS, Abaraogu UO. TENS and heat therapy for pain relief and quality of life improvement in individuals with primary dysmenorrhea: a systematic review. Complement Ther Clin Pract. 2016;24:86–91.
60. Proctor ML, Murphy PA, Pattison HM, et al. Behavioural interventions for primary and secondary dysmenorrhoea. Cochrane Database Syst Rev. 2007;(3):CD002248.
61. Proctor ML, Murphy PA. Herbal and dietary therapies for primary and secondary dysmenorrhoea. Cochrane Database Syst Rev. 2001;(3):CD002124.
62. Daily JW, Zhang X, Kim DS, Park S. Efficacy of ginger for alleviating the symptoms of primary dysmenorrhea: A systematic review and meta-analysis of randomized clinical trials. Pain Med. 2015;16(12):2243–55.
63. Chen CX, Barrett B, Kwekkeboom KL. Efficacy of oral ginger (*Zingiber officinale*) for dysmenorrhea: a systematic review and meta-analysis. Evid Based Complement Alternat Med. 2016;2016:6295737.
64. Ziaei S, Zakeri M, Kazemnejad A. A randomised controlled trial of vitamin E in the treatment of primary dysmenorrhoea. BJOG. 2005;112(4):466–9.
65. Mehrpooya M, Eshraghi A, Rabiee S, Larki-Harchegani A, Ataei S. Comparison of the effect of fish-oil and calcium supplementation on treatment of primary dysmenorrhea. Rev Recent Clin Trials. 2017;12(3):148–53.
66. Pattanittum P, Kunyanone N, Brown J, et al. Dietary supplements for dysmenorrhoea. Cochrane Database Syst Rev. 2016;(3):CD002124.
67. Israel RG, Sutton M, O'Brien KF. Effects of aerobic training on primary dysmenorrhea symptomatology in college females. J Am Coll Heal. 1985;33:241–4.
68. Brown J, Brown S. Exercise for dysmenorrhoea. Cochrane Database Syst Rev. 2010;(2):CD004142.
69. Golomb LM, Solidum AA, Warren MP. Primary dysmenorrhea and physical activity. Med Sci Sports Exerc. 1998;30:906–9.
70. Metheny WP, Smith RP. The relationship between exercise, stress, and primary dysmenorrhea. J Behav Med. 1989;12:569–86.
71. Rakhshaee Z. Effect of three yoga poses (cobra, cat and fish poses) in women with primary dysmenorrhea: a randomized clinical trial. J Pediatr Adolesc Gynecol. 2011;24:192–6.
72. Yang NY, Kim SD. Effects of a yoga program on menstrual cramps and menstrual distress in undergraduate students with primary dysmenorrhea: a single-blind, randomized controlled trial. J Altern Complement Med. 2016;22(9):732–8.
73. Hatcher RA. Counseling couples about coitus during menstrual flow. Contracept Technol Update. 1981;2:167.
74. Juang CM, Yen MS, Twu NF, Horng HC, Yu HC, Chen CY. Impact of pregnancy on primary dysmenorrhea. Int J Gynaecol Obstet. 2006;92(3):221–7.
75. Barnhart K, Furman I, Devoto L. Attitudes and practice of couples regarding sexual relations during the menses and spotting. Contraception. 1995;51(2):93–8.
76. Davis AR, Nowygrod S, Shabsigh R, Westhoff C. The influence of vaginal bleeding on the sexual behavior of urban, Hispanic women and men. Contraception. 2002;65(5):351–5.
77. Daley AJ. Exercise and primary dysmenorrhoea: a comprehensive and critical review of the literature. Sports Med. 2008;38(8):659–70.

78. Daley AJ. The role of exercise in the treatment of menstrual disorders: the evidence. Br J Gen Pract. 2009;59(561):241–2.
79. Fisher C, Sibbritt D, Hickman L, Adams JA. Critical review of complementary and alternative medicine use by women with cyclic perimenstrual pain and discomfort: a focus upon prevalence, patterns and applications of use and users' motivations, information seeking and self-perceived efficacy. Acta Obstet Gynecol Scand. 2016;95:861–71.
80. Armour M, Smith CA. Treating primary dysmenorrhoea with acupuncture: a narrative review of the relationship between acupuncture 'dose' and menstrual pain outcomes. Acupunct Med. 2016;34(6):416–24.
81. Liu CZ, Xie JP, Wang LP, et al. A randomized controlled trial of single point acupuncture in primary dysmenorrhea. Pain Med. 2014;15(6):910–20.
82. Smith CA, Armour M, Zhu X, et al. Acupuncture for dysmenorrhoea. Cochrane Database Syst Rev. 2016;(4):CD007854.
83. Wade C, Wang L, Zhao WJ, et al. Acupuncture point injection treatment of primary dysmenorrhoea: a randomised, double blind, controlled study. BMJ Open. 2016;6(1):e008166.
84. Yang M, Chen X, Bo L, et al. Moxibustion for pain relief in patients with primary dysmenorrhea: a randomized controlled trial. PLoS One. 2017;12(2):e0170952.
85. Gao J, Wang Q, Xian S, et al. The effect of moxibustion on alleviating menstrual pain in a population of young nursing students: a prospective randomized cross-over pilot study. Complement Ther Med. 2015;23(6):773–81.
86. Zhu X, Proctor M, Bensoussan A, et al. Chinese herbal medicine for primary dysmenorrhoea. Cochrane Database Syst Rev. 2007;(2):CD005288.
87. Pan JC, Tsai YT, Lai JN, Fang RC, Yeh CH. The traditional Chinese medicine prescription pattern of patients with primary dysmenorrhea in Taiwan: a large-scale cross sectional survey. J Ethnopharmacol. 2014;152(2):314–9.
88. Kokjohn K, Schmid DM, Triano JJ, Brennan PC. The effect of spinal manipulation on pain and prostaglandin levels in women with primary dysmenorrhea. J Manip Physiol Ther. 1992;15(5):279–85.
89. Proctor ML, Hing W, Johnson TC, Murphy PA. Spinal manipulation for primary and secondary dysmenorrhoea. Cochrane Database Syst Rev. 2006;(3):CD002119.
90. Hong GY, Shin BC, Park SN, et al. Randomized controlled trial of the efficacy and safety of self-adhesive low-level light therapy in women with primary dysmenorrhea. Int J Gynaecol Obstet. 2016;133(1):37–42.
91. Uysal M, Doğru HY, Sapmaz E, et al. Investigating the effect of rose essential oil in patients with primary dysmenorrhea. Complement Ther Clin Pract. 2016;24:45–9.
92. Shah M, Monga A, Patel S, Shah M, Bakshi H. The effect of hypnosis on dysmenorrhea. Int J Clin Exp Hypn. 2014;62(2):164–78.

Additional Resources

American College of Obstetricians and Gynecologists. Noncontraceptive uses of hormonal contraceptives. Practice Bulletin No. 110. Obstet Gynecol. 2010;115:206–18.
Anon. Drugs for pain. Treat Guidel Med Lett. 2013;11(128):31–42.
French L. Dysmenorrhea in adolescents: diagnosis and treatment. Paediatr Drugs. 2008;10(1):1–7.
Burnett M, Lemyre M. No. 345-primary dysmenorrhea consensus guideline. J Obstet Gynaecol Can. 2017;39(7):585–95.
Dawood MY. Dysmenorrhoea and prostaglandins: pharmacological and therapeutic considerations. Drugs. 1981;22(1):42–56.
Dawood MY. Nonsteroidal anti-inflammatory drugs and changing attitudes toward dysmenorrhea. Am J Med. 1988;84(5A):23–9.

Dawood MY. Primary dysmenorrhea: advances in pathogenesis and management. Obstet Gynecol. 2006;108(2):428–41.

Drugs for dysmenorrhea. Med Lett Drugs Ther. 1979;21(20):81–4.

Harel Z. Dysmenorrhea in adolescents. Ann N Y Acad Sci. 2008;1135:185–95.

Lefebvre G, Pinsonneault O, Antao V, et al. Primary dysmenorrhea consensus guideline. J Obstet Gynaecol Can. 2005;27(12):1117–46.

Latthe PM, Champaneria R, Khan KS. Dysmenorrhoea. BMJ Clin Evid. 2011;2011. pii: 0813.

Marjoribanks J, Proctor M, Farquhar C, Derks RS. Nonsteroidal anti-inflammatory drugs for dysmenorrhoea. Cochrane Database Syst Rev. 2010;(7):CD001751.

Proctor M, Farquhar C. Diagnosis and management of dysmenorrhoea. BMJ Clin Evid. 2007;2007. pii: 0813.

Ryan SA. The treatment of dysmenorrhea. Pediatr Clin N Am. 2017;64(2):331–42.

Sanfilippo J, Erb T. Evaluation and management of dysmenorrhea in adolescents. Clin Obstet Gynecol. 2008;51(2):257–67.

For a quick and general overview of many of the pathologies that cause secondary dysmenorrhea:
Smith RP. Netter's obstetrics & gynecology. 3rd ed. Philadelphia: Elsevier; 2017. p. 71–3.

Chapter 10
Management Strategies for Primary Menorrhagia

10.1 Topic Overview

Unlike primary dysmenorrhea, the managements of primary and secondary menorrhagia are often intertwined and complicated by the prevalence of difficult-to-identify secondary causes. When true primary menorrhagia is encountered, the same prostaglandin reduction strategies that work so well in primary dysmenorrhea work well for heavy menstrual bleeding. They also work well for many forms of secondary menorrhagia, raising the possibility that underlying pathologies may be missed if a careful assessment is not carried out before treatment, with equally careful monitoring after initiation. Treatment without such evaluation and care may miss symptoms of an easily corrected condition or neoplastic disease.

The most effective treatments for heavy menstrual bleeding will always be driven by the underlying pathophysiology. They should also be informed by the severity of the blood loss, associated symptoms or needs (contraception or fertility), medical comorbidities, and patient preferences. Some of the therapeutic options alter the normal mechanisms of blood clotting; therefore, awareness of any underlying risks for thromboembolic disease or coagulopathies must be maintained. When underlying anemia or iron deficits are present, they should be addressed as well [1].

Except in the case of first menstrual bleeding for girls with profound coagulopathies, heavy menstrual bleeding presents as a recurrent problem. By definition, acute (noncyclic) vaginal bleeding lies outside the definition of heavy menstrual bleeding (PALM-COEIN: AUB/HMB), and its management will not be discussed here. Also omitted are acquired or compensated blood dyscrasias, which are presumed to have been diagnosed and appropriately treated.

© Springer International Publishing AG 2018
R.P. Smith, *Dysmenorrhea and Menorrhagia*,
https://doi.org/10.1007/978-3-319-71964-1_10

10.2   Pharmacologic Therapies

Efforts to outline a set of evidence-based guidelines for the treatment of heavy bleeding have been made, but have encountered difficulties with the quality of the data available, or have become outdated as new treatment options have become available [2]. A meta-analysis of reported studies on nonsurgical interventions for heavy menstrual bleeding found that many of the reported trials were of less than ideal quality, with unclear risks of bias, small sample sizes, and poor study design [3]. The result was that the information gleaned was limited and of insufficient quality to derive guidance. Despite this, pharmacologic therapy remains the most appropriate initial treatment for almost all patients with heavy menstrual bleeding, regardless of cause.

Medical therapies that are effective and usually well tolerated include the levonorgestrel-releasing intrauterine system (LNG-IUS) and oral medications such as tranexamic acid, nonsteroidal anti-inflammatory drugs (e.g., mefenamic acid), and combined estrogen/progestogen contraceptives. Less frequently used as initial therapy, but also effective, are long-acting contraceptives such as depot medroxyprogesterone acetate (DMPA), implantable subcutaneous contraceptive rods, and other forms of combined hormonal contraceptives such as rings or patches. For patients with an underlying bleeding disorder (e.g., von Willebrand disease), an additional option is intranasal desmopressin [4]. In all cases, it is important that the patient be fully involved in the decision-making process [5] (Fig. 10.1).

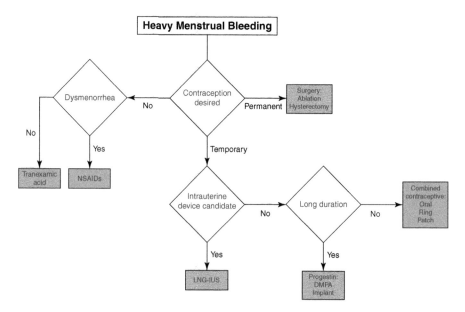

Fig. 10.1 One possible algorithm for the management of heavy menstrual bleeding. Some argue that even when permanent sterilization is desired, the levonorgestrel-releasing intrauterine system (LNG-IUS) is still a reasonable first step. *NSAIDs* nonsteroidal anti-inflammatory drugs, *DMPA* depot medroxyprogesterone acetate, *Implant* subdermal contraceptive implant

10.2.1 Hormonal Therapies

Many clinicians prefer to use hormonal treatments as first-line therapies for heavy menstrual bleeding of undocumented cause [6]. An attempt to perform a meta-analysis to determine the role of oral contraceptives versus other medical managements was unable to achieve its stated objectives because of the paucity of data [7]. In trials where menstrual blood loss has been actually measured, combination contraceptive formulations have shown significant reductions in flow, even to the point of returning patients to blood losses below the threshold of 80 mL [8–10] (Fig. 10.2).

A small study attempted to compare the therapeutic efficacies of norethisterone, tranexamic acid, and levonorgestrel-releasing intrauterine system for treating primary menorrhagia. The LNG-IUS was more effective than norethisterone and tranexamic acid in decreasing blood loss, but satisfaction rates and quality of life assessments across all groups were comparable [11]. Similar quality of life assessments have favored the use of the intrauterine system [12–15].

Because of convenience and efficacy, many have recommended the use of the levonorgestrel-releasing intrauterine system as first choice for patients not desiring pregnancy in the short term [16, 17]. When compared to oral medroxyprogesterone acetate, the LNG-IUS reduced menstrual blood loss more effectively and had a higher likelihood of treatment success [18–20]. The use of cyclic oral progestins has also been reported, but results show similar or inferior bleeding control to the LNG-IUS with less patient satisfaction [21, 22]. Data evaluating the efficacy of depot medroxyprogesterone acetate or the subdermal contraceptive implant is lacking, but the frequently encountered patient reports of "lighter" or absent menses associated with these methods would suggest they could be

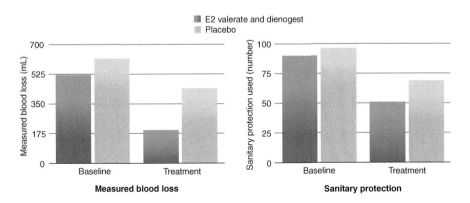

Fig. 10.2 Combination oral contraceptives have been shown to reduce measured blood loss and the number of items of sanitary protection used, as seen in this 2011 study by Jensen et al. [8]

Fig. 10.3 The
levonorgestrel-releasing
intrauterine system
contains between 13.5 and
52 mg of levonorgestrel
within a semipermeable
chamber, which is released
at a rate of roughly
14–20 mcg per day. This
release declines by from
1/2 to 2/3 over the
indicated life of the device

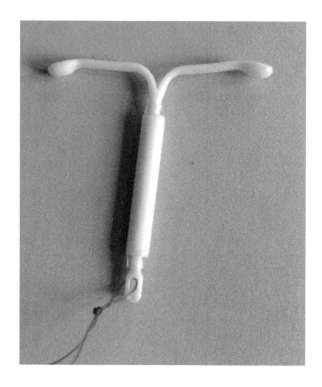

considered when the amount of bleeding is not excessive and cycle control is not an issue (Fig. 10.3).

Several studies have compared the LNG-IUS and combination oral contraceptives for their effectiveness in reducing heavy menstrual bleeding and have generally reported some degree of superiority for the intrauterine system [23, 24]. This finding has been supported in broader literature reviews [25]. A systematic review of 21 reported randomized controlled trials found that the LNG-IUS was superior to combined oral contraceptives in reducing menstrual blood loss [26]; however, cost-benefit analysis results recommend oral treatment as the first-line treatment for menorrhagia [27] because of the high initial cost of the LNG-IUS. This leaves the clinician at a loss for a definitive final choice based upon available evidence. It should be recognized that women who have significant pain with their heavy menses have a higher rate of discontinuation of intrauterine devices in general [28].

One reported trial suggests that both the contraceptive vaginal ring and contraceptive patch are very effective short-term treatments for heavy menstrual bleeding. There was better cycle control and compliance with the vaginal ring, making it a more attractive option for many women [29]. These findings are similar to pilot studies reported comparing the ring and oral contraceptives [30, 31]. Despite a statistically significant reduction in blood loss measured by a pictorial blood loss assessment chart, the reductions reported still left most of the participants within the range of heavy menstrual bleeding reported for these tools [32, 33]. Notwithstanding documented efficacy of hormonal contraceptives in reducing menstrual bleeding, providers must be sensitive to possible resistance to the use of these agents by some adolescent patients or their parents [34].

While suppression of the menstrual cycle by the use of gonadotropin-releasing hormone (GnRH) agonists or selective estrogen receptor modulators (SERMs), such as danazol, can be used to stop heavy menstrual blood loss, they are not appropriate for long-term use [35]. Experience with the novel option of selective progesterone receptor modulators in the treatment of heavy menstrual bleeding associated with uterine leiomyomata has been described [36], but they are not likely to play a large role in treating primary menorrhagia in the foreseeable future.

10.2.2 Nonsteroidal Anti-inflammatory Agents

Prostaglandin inhibitors have been found to decrease menstrual blood loss by 30–50% [37–39] while also relieving cramping (see Chap. 9). Mefenamic acid, specifically, has been used effectively for the control of long-standing heavy menstrual bleeding [40]. When compared with tranexamic acid and levonorgestrel-containing intrauterine devices, mefenamic acid significantly decreased menstrual blood loss [41], though this and other reviews have suggested that hormonal and other therapies may be superior [42]. For example, one meta-analysis concluded that NSAIDs, such as mefenamic acid, were less effective than the LNG-IUS or tranexamic acid in reducing menstrual bleeding [43]. It should be noted that despite this reported superiority, these studies still show that mefenamic acid and other NSAIDs are sufficiently effective to reduce menstrual blood loss, often back to below 80 mL per cycle [41], making the assertion of superiority moot. Accordingly, NSAIDs should still hold a place for the treatment of selected patients (Fig. 10.4).

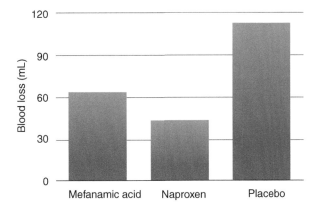

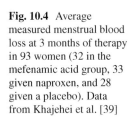

Fig. 10.4 Average measured menstrual blood loss at 3 months of therapy in 93 women (32 in the mefenamic acid group, 33 given naproxen, and 28 given a placebo). Data from Khajehei et al. [39]

10.2.3 Antifibrinolytics

Antifibrinolytic drugs, such as tranexamic acid, work by inhibiting fibrinolysis. Tranexamic acid is a synthetic lysine amino acid derivative, which reduces the plasmin dissolution of hemostatic fibrin. When tranexamic acid is present, the plasmin lysine receptor binding sites for fibrin become occupied, preventing binding with fibrin monomers, thus protecting and stabilizing fibrin's matrix structure [3].

These drugs reduce bleeding by about 40–60% [44–47] but do not generally alleviate menstrual cramping [48]. They are taken only during menstruation and are usually well tolerated but can cause mild nausea and diarrhea [49], headaches, sinus and nasal symptoms, back pain, abdominal pain, musculoskeletal pain, joint pain, muscle cramps, migraine, anemia, and fatigue. One small study attempted to evaluate oral tranexamic acid versus combined oral contraceptives for adolescent heavy menstrual bleeding and found them to comparable in terms of menstrual flow [50]. Because tranexamic acid is an antifibrinolytic, concomitant use of hormonal contraception may further increase the thrombotic risk associated with combination hormonal contraceptives [51]. Even without such rick factors, occasional incidents of drug-related thrombosis in tranexamic acid users have been reported [52].

At least one systematic review has found that tranexamic acid demonstrated consistent reductions in menstrual blood loss, and improvements in quality of life, when reported [53]. As has been demonstrated with NSAID therapy, the patients who garner the most benefit with tranexamic acid treatment are those who begin with the greatest blood loss [54] (Fig. 10.5).

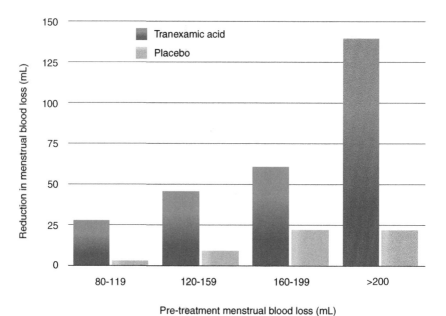

Fig. 10.5 The amount of improvement seen during treatment for heavy menstrual bleeding is often a function of the degree of hemorrhage, as seen in this data from 196 women randomized to receive tranexamic acid ($n = 123$) or placebo ($n = 73$). Data from LUKE et al. [54]

Desmopressin is a synthetic analog of vasopressin, which promotes the release of von Willebrand factor from endothelial cell storage sites. Its use is primarily for the management of patients with bleeding disorders who have acute bleeding episodes. A non-randomized comparison supported the value of combining desmopressin and tranexamic acid for bleeding in such patients. When tranexamic acid was compared to desmopressin, a single study showed better reduction in menstrual blood loss with tranexamic acid than with desmopressin [3].

10.2.4 Complementary and Alternative Therapies

Treatments advocated for excessive or insufficient menstrual bleeding have included many alternative approaches such as vibration therapy [55] or dietary changes [56]. As with dysmenorrhea treatments, small study sizes, differing study designs, varying routes of administration, and the range of herbal remedies tested have resulted in an inability to draw clinically useful conclusions [57, 58] (Fig. 10.6).

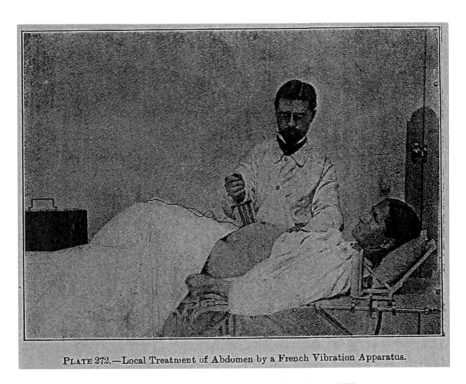

PLATE 272.—Local Treatment of Abdomen by a French Vibration Apparatus.

Fig. 10.6 A 1902 illustration of the use of abdominal vibration therapy [55]

10.3   Surgical Options

In the United States, menstrual bleeding disorders are a leading indication for hysterectomy [59]. The most common causes of secondary menorrhagia are uterine leiomyomas or adenomyosis, which are often treated with surgery. Medical management still represents appropriate initial treatment for these patients. Older surgical approaches, such as dilatation and curettage, have either not been studied against another treatment or have been found to have little effect beyond the first month following the procedure [2].

Women frequently choose surgical therapy following intermediate to long-term medical therapy. A systematic review of available trials of women with heavy menstrual bleeding found that 59% of women randomized to oral medications had had surgery within 2 years and 77% within 5 years [60]. Similarly, by 10 years, 46% of women originally assigned to a hormone-releasing intrauterine device had undergone hysterectomy.

The lack of long-term efficacy is a problem with any medical management that must be continued for a good proportion of a woman's reproductive life. For example, one randomized trial followed 63 women with persistent menstrual dysfunction and monitored to see if they underwent hysterectomy or switched medical therapy [61]. By 18 months, 53% of women in the medical treatment group had undergone hysterectomy (median interval was 6 months). In another trial of uterine artery ligation via minilaparotomy in 30 women, 20% (6/30) underwent hysterectomy within 12 months [62]. A cost analysis found that at 2 years, mean costs expended in medical management and hysterectomy cohorts were $4479 and $6777, respectively [63]. Broken down to resource use by treatment received, the costs for medication only, medicine followed by hysterectomy, and hysterectomy only were $2595, $6128, and $7024, respectively. These findings have been replicated in other analyses [64, 65], underscoring the desirability of and least an initial trial of medical management.

Endometrial resection or ablation offers a less invasive option to hysterectomy for some patients: After 4 months, endometrial resection was significantly more effective than oral medication in controlling bleeding (odds ratio [OR] 10.6, 95% CI 5.3–21.3) and significantly less likely to cause side effects (OR 0.2, 95% CI 0.1–0.3) [60]. However, for women with heavy bleeding due to adenomyosis, endometrial ablation may be less effective than in other conditions. With any ablative technique, there is no guarantee that bleeding will be reduced to acceptable levels in the long term. In one study, after 4 years, 38% of those who had had endometrial resection went on to receive further surgical treatment of some kind for continued symptoms [66]. This potential need for re-treatment narrows the cost gap between hysterectomy and conservative surgery [67]. A Cochrane systematic review has found that success rates and complication profiles of newer techniques of ablation (e.g., heat, cold, microwave, or other forms of energy) appear to compare favorably with older hysteroscopic techniques [68], though many reports do not quantify the improvement in bleeding [69, 70].

Key Points

- The treatment of heavy menstrual bleeding without clinically identified cause (primary menorrhagia) is often the same as the initial treatment used as an alternative to definitive management in cases of identified pathology (e.g., uterine leiomyomas).
- Because many of the available treatments for heavy menstrual bleeding will work well in the early stages of significant pathologies (e.g., endometrial hyperplasia or cancer, endometrial polyps, uterine leiomyomata, etc.), a careful evaluation must be carried out prior to instituting treatment.
- Except for those actively pursuing pregnancy or in whom an intrauterine device is contraindicated, the levonorgestrel-releasing intrauterine system (LNG-IUS) has become the initial treatment of choice for many patients.
- Treatment with nonsteroidal anti-inflammatory drugs (NSAIDs) can be especially effective for those women who suffer menstrual pain along with their excessive bleeding.
- Antifibrinolytic medications are an effective alternative to hormonal or anti-cyclooxygenase treatments for selected patients.

References

1. Peuranpää P, Heliövaara-Peippo S, Fraser I, Paavonen J, Hurskainen R. Effects of anemia and iron deficiency on quality of life in women with heavy menstrual bleeding. Acta Obstet Gynecol Scand. 2014;93(7):654–60.
2. Royal New Zealand College of Obstetricians and Gynaecologists, Royal New Zealand College of General Practitioners. An evidence-based guideline for the management of heavy menstrual bleeding. Working Party for Guidelines for the Management of Heavy Menstrual Bleeding. N Z Med J. 1999;112(1088):174–7.
3. Ray S, Ray A. Non-surgical interventions for treating heavy menstrual bleeding (menorrhagia) in women with bleeding disorders. Cochrane Database Syst Rev. 2014;(11):CD010338.
4. Fraser IS, Porte RJ, Kouides PA, Lukes AS. A benefit-risk review of systemic haemostatic agents: part 2: in excessive or heavy menstrual bleeding. Drug Saf. 2008;31(4):275–82.
5. Zandstra D, Busser JA, Aarts JW, Nieboer TE. Interventions to support shared decision-making for women with heavy menstrual bleeding: a systematic review. Eur J Obstet Gynecol Reprod Biol. 2017;211:156–63.
6. Heikinheimo O, Fraser I. The current status of hormonal therapies for heavy menstrual bleeding. Best Pract Res Clin Obstet Gynaecol. 2017;40:111–20.
7. Farquhar C, Brown J. Oral contraceptive pill for heavy menstrual bleeding. Cochrane Database Syst Rev. 2009;(4):CD000154.
8. Jensen JT, Parke S, Mellinger U, Machlitt A, Fraser IS. Effective treatment of heavy menstrual bleeding with estradiol valerate and dienogest: a randomized controlled trial. Obstet Gynecol. 2011;117(4):777–87.
9. Fraser IS, Parke S, Mellinger U, Machlitt A, Serrani M, Jensen J. Effective treatment of heavy and/or prolonged menstrual bleeding without organic cause: pooled analysis of two multinational, randomised, double-blind, placebo-controlled trials of oestradiol valerate and dienogest. Eur J Contracept Reprod Health Care. 2011;16(4):258–69.
10. Fraser IS, Jensen J, Schaefers M, Mellinger U, Parke S, Serrani M. Normalization of blood loss in women with heavy menstrual bleeding treated with an oral contraceptive containing estradiol valerate/dienogest. Contraception. 2012;86(2):96–101.

11. Kiseli M, Kayikcioglu F, Evliyaoglu O, Haberal A. Comparison of therapeutic efficacies of norethisterone, tranexamic acid and levonorgestrel-releasing intrauterine system for the treatment of heavy menstrual bleeding: a randomized controlled study. Gynecol Obstet Investig. 2016;81(5):447–53.
12. Heliövaara-Peippo S, Hurskainen R, Teperi J, et al. Quality of life and costs of levonorgestrel-releasing intrauterine system or hysterectomy in the treatment of menorrhagia: a 10-year randomized controlled trial. Am J Obstet Gynecol. 2013;209(6):535.e1–14.
13. Xu L, Lee BS, Asif S, Kraemer P, Inki P. Satisfaction and health-related quality of life in women with heavy menstrual bleeding; results from a non-interventional trial of the levonorgestrel-releasing intrauterine system or conventional medical therapy. Int J Womens Health. 2014;6:547–54.
14. Sanghera S, Roberts TE, Barton P, et al. Levonorgestrel-releasing intrauterine system vs. usual medical treatment for menorrhagia: an economic evaluation alongside a randomised controlled trial. PLoS One. 2014;9(3):e91891.
15. Matteson KA, Rahn DD, Wheeler TL 2nd, et al. Society of Gynecologic Surgeons Systematic Review Group. Nonsurgical management of heavy menstrual bleeding: a systematic review. Obstet Gynecol. 2013;121(3):632–43.
16. Uhm S, Perriera L. Hormonal contraception as treatment for heavy menstrual bleeding: a systematic review. Clin Obstet Gynecol. 2014;57(4):694–717.
17. Bitzer J, Heikinheimo O, Nelson AL, Calaf-Alsina J, Fraser IS. Medical management of heavy menstrual bleeding: a comprehensive review of the literature. Obstet Gynecol Surv. 2015;70(2):115–30.
18. Kaunitz AM, Bissonnette F, Monteiro I, Lukkari-Lax E, Muysers C, Jensen JT. Levonorgestrel-releasing intrauterine system or medroxyprogesterone for heavy menstrual bleeding: a randomized controlled trial. Obstet Gynecol. 2010;116(3):625–32.
19. Kaunitz AM, Bissonnette F, Monteiro I, Lukkari-Lax E, DeSanctis Y, Jensen J. Levonorgestrel-releasing intrauterine system for heavy menstrual bleeding improves hemoglobin and ferritin levels. Contraception. 2012;86(5):452–7.
20. Kaunitz AM, Inki P. The levonorgestrel-releasing intrauterine system in heavy menstrual bleeding: a benefit-risk review. Drugs. 2012;72(2):193–215.
21. Hurskainen R, Grenman S, Komi I, et al. Diagnosis and treatment of menorrhagia. Acta Obstet Gynecol Scand. 2007;86(6):749–57.
22. Lethaby A, Irvine G, Cameron I. Cyclical progestogens for heavy menstrual bleeding. Cochrane Database Syst Rev. 2008;(1):CD001016.
23. Shaaban MM, Zakherah MS, El-Nashar SA, Sayed GH. Levonorgestrel-releasing intrauterine system compared to low dose combined oral contraceptive pills for idiopathic menorrhagia: a randomized clinical trial. Contraception. 2011;83(1):48–54.
24. Lee BS, Ling X, Asif S, Kraemer P, Hanisch JU, Inki P. Levonorgestrel-releasing intrauterine system versus conventional medical therapy for heavy menstrual bleeding in the Asia-Pacific region. Int J Gynaecol Obstet. 2013;121(1):24–30.
25. Qiu J, Cheng J, Wang Q, Hua J. Levonorgestrel-releasing intrauterine system versus medical therapy for menorrhagia: a systematic review and meta-analysis. Med Sci Monit. 2014;20:1700–13.
26. Lethaby A, Hussain M, Rishworth JR, Rees MC. Progesterone or progestogen-releasing intrauterine systems for heavy menstrual bleeding. Cochrane Database Syst Rev. 2015;(4):CD002126.
27. Sanghera S, Frew E, Gupta JK, Kai J, Roberts TE. Exploring the use of cost-benefit analysis to compare pharmaceutical treatments for menorrhagia. PharmacoEconomics. 2015;33(9):957–65.
28. Maguire K, Joslin-Roher S, Westhoff CL, Davis AR. IUDs at 1 year: predictors of early discontinuation. Contraception. 2015;92(6):575–7.
29. Dahiya P, Dalal M, Yadav A, Dahiya K, Jain S, Silan V. Efficacy of combined hormonal vaginal ring in comparison to combined hormonal pills in heavy menstrual bleeding. Eur J Obstet Gynecol Reprod Biol. 2016;203:147–51.

30. Abu Hashim H, Alsherbini W, Bazeed M. Contraceptive vaginal ring treatment of heavy menstrual bleeding: a randomized controlled trial with norethisterone. Contraception. 2012;85(3):246–52.
31. Agarwal N, Gupta M, Kriplani A, Bhatla N, Singh N. Comparison of combined hormonal vaginal ring with ultralow-dose combined oral contraceptive pills in the management of heavy menstrual bleeding: a pilot study. J Obstet Gynaecol. 2016;36(1):71–5.
32. Janssen CA, Scholten PC, Heintz APA. Simple visual assessment technique to discriminate between menorrhagia and normal menstrual blood loss. Obstet Gynecol. 1995;85(6):977–82.
33. Zakherah MS, Sayed GH, El-Nashar SA, Shaaban MM. Pictorial blood loss assessment chart in the evaluation of heavy menstrual bleeding: diagnostic accuracy compared with alkaline hematin. Gynecol Obstet Investig. 2011;71(4):281–4.
34. Yiu KW, Chan SS, Chung TK. Mothers' attitude to the use of a combined oral contraceptive pill by their daughters for menstrual disorders or contraception. Hong Kong Med J. 2017;23(2):150–7.
35. Agarwal N, Kriplani A. Medical management of dysfunctional uterine bleeding. Int J Gynecol Obstet. 2001;75(2):199–201.
36. Maybin JA, Critchley HO. Medical management of heavy menstrual bleeding. Womens Health (Lond). 2016;12(1):27–34.
37. Hall P, Maclachlan N, Horn N, Nudd MWE, Taylor CG, Garrioch DB. Control of menorrhagia by the cyclo-oxygenase inhibitors naproxen sodium and mefenamic acid. Br J Obstet Gynaecol. 1987;94:554–8.
38. van Eijkeren MA, Christiaens GC, Geuze HJ, Haspels AA, Sixma JJ. Effects of mefenamic acid on menstrual haemostasis in essential menorrhagia. Am J Obstet Gynecol. 1992;166(5):1419–28.
39. Khajehei M, Abdali K, Tabatabaee H. The effect of mefenamic acid and naproxen on heavy menstrual bleeding: a placebo-controlled study. S Afr J OG. 2013;19(2):31–4.
40. Fraser IS, McCarron G, Markham R, Robinson M, Smyth E. Long-term treatment of menorrhagia with mefenamic acid. Obstet Gynecol. 1983;61(1):3–6.
41. Reid PC, Virtanen-Kari S. Randomised comparative trial of the levonorgestrel intrauterine system and mefenamic acid for the treatment of idiopathic menorrhagia: a multiple analysis using total menstrual fluid loss, menstrual blood loss and pictorial blood loss assessment charts. Br J Obstet Gynecol. 2005;112(8):8–14.
42. Coulter A, Long A, Kelland J, et al. Managing menorrhagia. Qual Health Care. 1995;4(3):218–26.
43. Lethaby A, Duckitt K, Farquhar C. Non-steroidal anti-inflammatory drugs for heavy menstrual bleeding. Cochrane Database Syst Rev. 2013;(1):CD000400.
44. Bonner J, Sheppard BL. Treatment of menorrhagia during menstruation: randomized controlled trial of ethamsylate, mefenamic acid, and tranexamic acid. BMJ. 1996;313:579–82.
45. Lethaby A, Farquhar C, Cooke I. Antifibrinolytics for heavy menstrual bleeding. Cochrane Database Syst Rev. 2000;(4):CD000249.
46. Philipp CS. Antifibrinolytics in women with menorrhagia. Thromb Res. 2011;127(Suppl 3):S113–5.
47. Leminen H, Hurskainen R. Tranexamic acid for the treatment of heavy menstrual bleeding: efficacy and safety. Int J Womens Health. 2012;4:413–21.
48. Preston JT, Cameron IT, Adams EJ, Smith SK. Comparative study of tranexamic acid and norethisterone in the treatment of ovulatory menorrhagia. Br J Obstet Gynaecol. 1995;102:401–6.
49. Dunn CJ, Goa KL. Tranexamic acid: a review of its use in surgery and other indications. Drugs. 1999;57(6):1005–32.
50. Srivaths LV, Dietrich JE, Yee DL, Sangi-Haghpeykar H, Mahoney D Jr. Oral tranexamic acid versus combined oral contraceptives for adolescent heavy menstrual bleeding: a pilot study. J Pediatr Adolesc Gynecol. 2015;28(4):254–7.
51. Iacobellis G, Iacobellis G. Combined treatment with tranexamic acid and oral contraceptive pill causes coronary ulcerated plaque and acute myocardial infarction. Cardiovasc Drugs Ther. 2004;18(3):239–40.

52. Wijetilleka S, Yeo DCM, Sharma B. Central retinal artery occlusion in a 30-year-old woman taking tranexamic acid. BMJ Case Rep. 2017 July 13;2017. pii: bcr-2016-218246.
53. Edlund M. Nonhormonal treatments for heavy menstrual bleeding. J Womens Health (Larchmt). 2011;20(11):1645–53.
54. Lukes AS, Moore KA, Muse KN, et al. Tranexamic acid treatment for heavy menstrual bleeding: a randomized controlled trial. Obstet Gynecol. 2010;116(4):865–75.
55. Monell SH. A system of instruction in X-ray methods and medical uses of light, hot-air, vibration and high-frequency currents: a pictorial system of teaching by clinical instruction plates with explanatory text: a series of photographic clinics in standard uses of scientific therapeutic apparatus for surgical and medical practitioners: prepared especially for the post-graduate home study of surgeons, general physicians, dentists, dermatologists and specialists in the treatment of chronic diseases, and sanitarium practice. New York: E.R. Pelton; 1902, plate 372.
56. Kashefi F, Khajehei M, Alavinia M, Golmakani E, Asili J. Effect of ginger (Zingiber officinale) on heavy menstrual bleeding: a placebo-controlled, randomized clinical trial. Phytother Res. 2015;29(1):114–9.
57. Javan R, Yousefi M, Nazari SM, et al. Herbal medicines in idiopathic heavy menstrual bleeding: a systematic review. Phytother Res. 2016;30(10):1584–91.
58. Tansaz M, Memarzadehzavareh H, Qaraaty M, Eftekhar T, Tabarrai M, Kamalinejad M. Menorrhagia management in Iranian traditional medicine. J Evid Based Complement Altern Med. 2016;21(1):71–6.
59. Farquhar C, Steiner C. Hysterectomy rates in the United States 1990–1997. Obstet Gynecol. 2002;99:229–34.
60. Marjoribanks J, Lethaby A, Farquhar C. Surgery versus medical therapy for heavy menstrual bleeding. Cochrane Database Syst Rev. 2016;(1):CD003855.
61. Kuppermann M, Varner RE, Summitt RL Jr, et al. Effect of hysterectomy vs medical treatment on health-related quality of life and sexual functioning: the medicine or surgery (Ms) randomized trial. JAMA. 2004;291:1447–55.
62. Hassanin IM, Shahin AY, Abdel-Hafeez AT, Salem HT, El-Nashar SA. Bilateral uterine artery ligation via minilaparotomy for heavy menstrual bleeding. Int J Gynaecol Obstet. 2008;103(3):222–6.
63. Showstack J, Lin F, Learman LA, et al. Randomized trial of medical treatment versus hysterectomy for abnormal uterine bleeding: resource use in the medicine or surgery (Ms) trial. Am J Obstet Gynecol. 2006;194:332–8.
64. Learman LA, Summitt RL Jr, Varner RE, et al. Hysterectomy versus expanded medical treatment for abnormal uterine bleeding: clinical outcomes in the medicine or surgery trial. Obstet Gynecol. 2004;103:824–33.
65. Brown PM, Farquhar CM, Lethaby A, Sadler LC, Johnson NP. Cost-effectiveness analysis of levonorgestrel intrauterine system and thermal balloon ablation for heavy menstrual bleeding. BJOG. 2006;113(7):797–803.
66. Aberdeen Endometrial Ablation Trials Group. A randomised trial of endometrial ablation versus hysterectomy for the treatment of dysfunctional uterine bleeding: outcome at four years. Aberdeen Endometrial Ablation Trials Group. Br J Obstet Gynaecol. 1999;106(4):360–6.
67. Fergusson RJ, Lethaby A, Shepperd S, Farquhar C. Endometrial resection and ablation versus hysterectomy for heavy menstrual bleeding. Cochrane Database Syst Rev. 2013;(11):CD000329.
68. Daniels JP, Middleton LJ, Champaneria R, et al. International Heavy Menstrual Bleeding IPD Meta-analysis Collaborative Group. Second generation endometrial ablation techniques for heavy menstrual bleeding: network meta-analysis. BMJ. 2012;344:e2564.
69. Vihko KK, Raitala R, Taina E. Endometrial thermoablation for treatment of menorrhagia: comparison of two methods in outpatient setting. Acta Obstet Gynecol Scand. 2003;82(3):269–74.
70. Al-Shaikh G, Almalki G, Bukhari M, Fayed A, Al-Mandeel H. Effectiveness and outcomes of thermablate endometrial ablation system in women with heavy menstrual bleeding. J Obstet Gynaecol. 2017;37(6):770–4.

Additional Resources

American College of Obstetricians and Gynecologists. Endometrial ablation. ACOG Practice Bulletin No. 81. Obstet Gynecol. 2007;109:1233–48.

American College of Obstetricians and Gynecologists. Alternatives to hysterectomy in the management of leiomyomas. ACOG Practice Bulletin No. 96. Obstet Gynecol. 2008;112:201–7.

American College of Obstetricians and Gynecologists. Noncontraceptive uses of hormonal contraceptives. Practice Bulletin No. 110. Obstet Gynecol. 2010;115:206–18.

American College of Obstetricians and Gynecologists. Management of abnormal uterine bleeding associated with ovulatory dysfunction. Practice Bulletin No. 136. Obstet Gynecol. 2013;122:176–85.

American College of Obstetricians and Gynecologists. Management of acute abnormal uterine bleeding in nonpregnant reproductive-aged women. Committee Opinion No. 557. Obstet Gynecol. 2013;121:891–6.

American College of Obstetricians and Gynecologists. Von Willebrand disease in women. Committee Opinion No. 580. Obstet Gynecol. 2013;122:1368–73.

American College of Obstetricians and Gynecologists. Options for prevention and management of heavy menstrual bleeding in adolescent patients undergoing cancer treatment. Committee Opinion No. 606. Obstet Gynecol. 2014;124:397–402.

Bradley LD, Gueye NA. The medical management of abnormal uterine bleeding in reproductive-aged women. Am J Obstet Gynecol. 2016;214(1):31–44.

Davies J, Kadir RA. Heavy menstrual bleeding: an update on management. Thromb Res. 2017;151(Suppl 1):S70–7.

Fraser IS, Zeun S, Parke S, Wilke B, Junge W, Serrani M. Improving the objective quality of large-scale clinical trials for women with heavy menstrual bleeding: experience from 2 multi-center, randomized trials. Reprod Sci. 2013;20(7):745–54.

Kumar V, Chodankar R, Gupta JK. Endometrial ablation for heavy menstrual bleeding. Womens Health (Lond). 2016;12(1):45–52.

Leebeek FW, Eikenboom JC. Von Willebrand's disease. N Engl J Med. 2016;375(21):2067–80.

Mishell DR Jr, Fisher HW, Haynes PJ, Jones GS, Smith RP. Menorrhagia: a symposium. J Reprod Med. 1984;29(10 Suppl):763–82.

Oehler MK, Rees MC. Menorrhagia: an update. Acta Obstet Gynecol Scand. 2003;82(5):405–22.

Rodeghiero F. Management of menorrhagia in women with inherited bleeding disorders: general principles and use of desmopressin. Haemophilia. 2008;14(Suppl 1):21–30.

Smith RP. Netter's obstetrics & gynecology. 3rd ed. Philadelphia: Elsevier; 2017. p. 274–6.

Wellington K, Wagstaff AJ. Tranexamic acid: a review of its use in the management of menorrhagia. Drugs. 2003;63:1417–33.

Chapter 11
Options for When Simple Managements Are Not Enough

11.1 Topic Overview

Both menstrual pain and heavy menstrual bleeding no longer represent the debilitating threat they once posed. Inexpensive, safe, effective non-prescription therapy available without medical consultation means that dysmenorrhea is no longer the source of disability it once was. When this is not enough, prescription interventions offer exceptional efficacy. When heavy menstrual bleeding is experienced, the placement of a hormone-releasing intrauterine device (LNG-IUS) offers efficacy for 5 or more years with no further actions by the user. Normality can be restored, worry relieved, and function maintained.

Unfortunately, therapeutic failures may be as high as 20–25% of cases [1]. It is for these women that the skills of the clinician are required to achieve normal function. It is reasonable to expect that even in these cases, improvement is possible using care, therapeutic combinations, and more aggressive options.

11.2 Reassessing the Current Treatment

Because of the documented efficacy of most treatments for dysmenorrhea or heavy menstrual bleeding, the first step in managing any treatment failure must be a reassessment of the original diagnosis: Women who do not achieve adequate pain relief with nonsteroidal anti-inflammatory drugs (NSAIDs) and hormonal contraceptives may have secondary dysmenorrhea; women whose blood loss appears to continue may have endometrial pathology or leiomyomata. Once this diagnostic reassessment has occurred, a reassessment and modification of the treatment plan may be entertained (Fig. 11.1).

© Springer International Publishing AG 2018
R.P. Smith, *Dysmenorrhea and Menorrhagia*,
https://doi.org/10.1007/978-3-319-71964-1_11

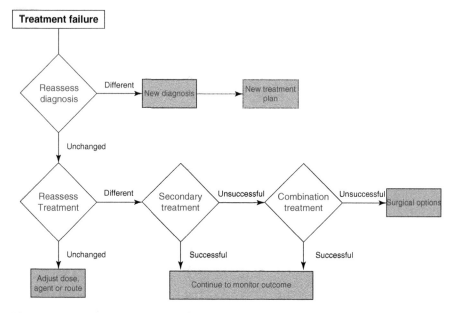

Fig. 11.1 One possible approach to failed treatments for dysmenorrhea or heavy menstrual bleeding

11.2.1 Dysmenorrhea

Once an NSAID has been selected, it should be tried over two to four menstrual cycles before success or failure can be assessed. If this initial therapy is unsuccessful, some patients may still have favorable response to another NSAID. For the best chance of success, this second drug should be chosen from a different chemical class (see Chap. 7). Patients should be reminded to take their medication at, or just before, the start of menstruation or symptoms. They should maintain consistent dosing for as long as symptoms would normally have lasted had medication not been used—for most patients, this will be 2–3 days.

Care should be taken in discounting the effectiveness of NSAID therapy based on a patient's experience with over-the-counter preparations. With the availability of non-prescription strengths of the agents, many patients may report having tried one or more without success. Some of these failures may only represent inadequate dosage. For example, non-prescription ibuprofen is 200 mg per tablet with a maximum daily dosage of 1200 mg, while many patients require an initial dose of 1200–1600 mg, followed by between 600 and 800 mg doses. Though some patients will obtain relief simply by increasing the dosage, many patients prefer to try "a different medication." Pharmacology aside, it is sometimes therapeutic to defer to the patient's wishes and change medications. When pain relief is not complete, patients should be warned not to add additional analgesics, especially NSAIDs, because of additive gastrointestinal and other side effects. The addition of caffeine ($\geq$100 mg) to a standard dose of commonly used analgesics provides a small but important increase in the proportion of participants who experience good pain relief [2].

To avoid the incremental or increased incidence of side effects associated with either adding additional analgesics or moving to stronger agents, changing to or adding different treatment modalities is reasonable. Both transcutaneous electrical nerve stimulation (TENS) and topical low-level heat have demonstrated efficacy, will not interfere with NSAID action, and will not potentiate side effects. The two modalities may even be combined with each other [3, 4].

As long as there are no immediate plans for conception, reducing endometrial prostaglandin production by thinning the endometrium is another option. This may be accomplished using either combination estrogen/progesterone contraceptives (oral, or less often, ring or patch) or intrauterine progestins, using the levonorgestrel-releasing intrauterine system (LNG-IUS). For many women, the addition of contraception is a welcome benefit, but for others it is not [5]. It should be noted that some studies of the contraceptive patch in adolescents have actually reported a roughly 10% chance of worsening menstrual pain (versus a roughly 40% improvement) [6].

Depot medroxyprogesterone acetate injections may also be used to suppress menstruation but provide a greater risk of breakthrough bleeding. Since this drug has been linked to concerns regarding its effect on bone mineral density, care should be used when considering its use during adolescence, a critical period for bone accrual (Fig. 11.2).

When cramps persist despite what should have been effective therapy, a wide-ranging reassessment is indicated. In adolescents especially, the reappraisal should include discussion of family, school, and other potential sources of stress, worsening the perception of pain. The potential of abuse, physical, emotional, or sexual, should be considered. The presence of "secondary agendas," such as emerging sexuality, sexual identity, or the need for contraception that cannot be directly voiced, can underlie the need for follow-up of a more acceptable complaint.

The likelihood of occult pelvic pathology is high among women with failed dysmenorrhea therapies. One study of 100 women with pelvic pain who did not have adequate pain relief with NSAIDs (some also treated with oral contraceptives)

WARNING: LOSS OF BONE MINERAL DENSITY

See full prescribing infromation for complete boxed warning.

• Women who use Depo-Provera Contraceptive Injection may lose significant bone mineral density. Bone loss is greater with increasing duration of use and may not be completely reversible.
• It is unknown if use of Depo-Provera Contraceptive Injection during adolescenece or early adulthood, a critical period of bone accretion, will reduce peak bone mass and increase the risk for osteoporotic fracture in later life.
• Depo-Provera Contraceptive Injection should not be used as a long-term birth control method (i.e., longer than 2 years) unless other birth control methods are considered inadequate.

Fig. 11.2 The current "Black Box Warning" required by the FDA to accompany the prescribing information for depot medroxyprogesterone acetate (Depo-Provera)

Fig. 11.3 Laparoscopic
view of pelvic adhesions
due to endometriosis, with
endometrial implants
visible over the bowel and
posterior cul-de-sac. Even
moderate involvement may
not be apparent on physical
examination

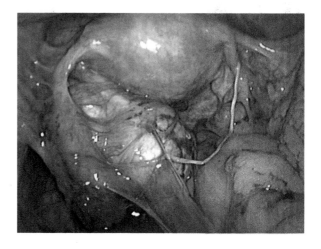

found that approximately 80% had endometriosis at laparoscopy [7]. Given this, diagnostic laparoscopy of women with failure with NSAIDs and oral contraceptive treatments is justifiable [8]. Intrauterine progestin delivery systems (LNG-IUS) have demonstrated some efficacy in women with dysmenorrhea secondary to either proven or suspected endometriosis (Fig. 11.3).

11.2.2 Menorrhagia

Because initial hormonal therapy, especially with the LNG-IUS, is both effective and targeted toward the end organ, when this treatment of heavy menstrual bleeding fails, there are often fewer remaining options. If the LNG-IUS has not been the first treatment, switching to this is reasonable. Suppressing menstruation with long-cycle oral contraceptives has been shown to be acceptable to many patients [9, 10] and provides fewer periods or absent bleeding. Depot medroxyprogesterone acetate may also be used in the same way, but cycle control is often poorer and side effects more common. Gonadotropin-releasing hormone (GnRH) agonists provide complete suppression of the hypothalamic-pituitary-ovarian axis, stopping menstruation, but are reserved for short-term use for specific pathologies, such as before surgical treatment of uterine leiomyomata. While less effective as an initial treatment than the LNG-IUS, the addition of an NSAID or tranexamic acid may still be appropriate.

11.3 Surgical Options

The ultimate surgical option for menstrual pain or heavy bleeding is hysterectomy. While definitive, this is clearly not the first choice for most women. Despite a natural reluctance to move to surgical options, especially in young women, there remains a place for surgery for both diagnosis and therapy in recalcitrant cases of dysmenorrhea or heavy menstrual bleeding.

11.3.1 Dysmenorrhea

Laparoscopic uterine nerve ablation has been proposed as a treatment for refractory dysmenorrhea for a number of years [11, 12]. A systematic review of two trials ($n = 68$ patients) found some evidence of the effectiveness of laparoscopic uterine nerve ablation (LUNA) for menstrual pain when measured at 12 months versus untreated controls (OR 6.12, 95% CI 1.78–21.03) [13]. Short-term effects at 6 months and quality of life assessments at 12 months were similar for both groups. This paucity of compelling data has been born out in subsequent reviews [14]. The wide confidence intervals and lack of long-term improvement in quality of life indicate that the efficacy of this surgical approach is uncertain, leading to the lack of support for this as a reliable treatment (Fig. 11.4).

At least one study has suggested that LUNA can be a useful adjunct in the treatment of symptomatic uterine leiomyomata. Among women undergoing uterine vessel coagulation for leiomyomata, the addition of uterine nerve ablation resulted in improved menstrual pain symptoms over 6-month follow-up [16]. However, when LUNA was compared to laparoscopic presacral neurectomy (LPSN) for pain, patients undergoing this procedure were significantly more likely to have pain relief at 12 months. LUNA combined with presacral neurectomy is not more effective than LUNA alone [17]. For both LUNA and LPSN, observational series have shown that success rates declined rapidly over time (years), possibly due to regrowth of nerves or pain signals being transferred via alternative routes [18, 19]. More evidence is needed before these procedures can be recommended.

11.3.2 Heavy Menstrual Bleeding

Because many causes of secondary menorrhagia are difficult to diagnose by simple history and physical means, failure to obtain the expected improvements in menstrual bleeding should suggest the possibility of pathology. The availability of simple-to-perform office-based hysteroscopy makes this an appropriate initial evaluation method when the diagnosis must be reassessed [20]. Some argue that performing hysteroscopy in a setting that allows conversion to operative procedures can save a step, combining diagnosis and therapy into a single step [21–23]. This decision should be driven by the experience of the clinician, the availability of appropriate instrumentation, the probability of pathology (and type), and the wishes of the patient [24, 25] (Fig. 11.5).

An alternative to removal of the uterus is the ablation or resection of the endometrial lining. Once again, depending on the equipment available and the experi-

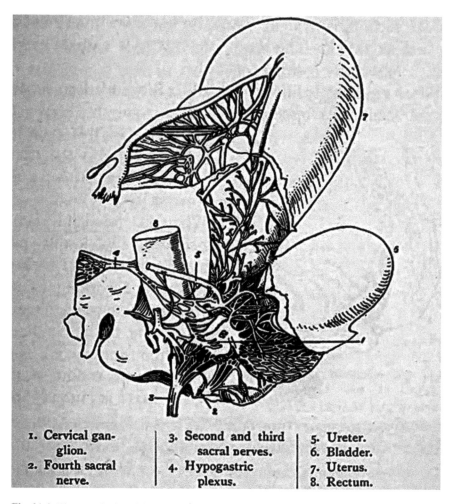

1. Cervical gan-glion.	3. Second and third sacral nerves.	5. Ureter.
2. Fourth sacral nerve.	4. Hypogastric plexus.	6. Bladder.
		7. Uterus.
		8. Rectum.

Fig. 11.4 The complexity of the uterine innervation can be seen in this 1898 illustration [15]. This complexity makes it very difficult to surgically interrupt all sensation from this organ

ence of the clinician, ablation can be performed in the office setting [27]. As noted in Chap. 10, not all patients will experience complete symptom relief, but for those who wish to retain their uterus and are nearing menopause, it may be a reasonable alternative [28, 29].

When the patient's symptoms are likely secondary to uterine leiomyomata, uterine artery embolization, focused ultrasonic or radiofrequency energy, and other techniques have been suggested as alternatives to hysterectomy for fibroids [30]. When heavy menstrual bleeding is associated with adenomyosis, there are currently no surgical alternatives to hysterectomy. A proof-of-concept study in 15 patients to evaluate the laparoscopic use of a "starburst" electrode to deliver radiofrequency energy to cause thermal ablation of adenomyosis has been reported [31].

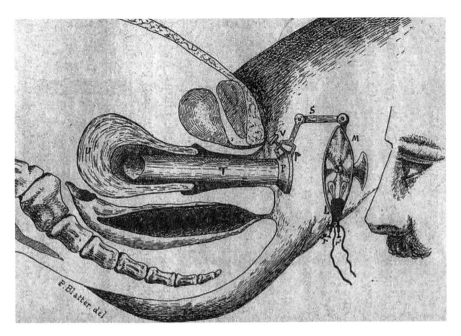

Fig. 11.5 Hysteroscopy as described by Duplay and Clado, in 1898, in the first book concerning hysteroscopy [26]

Key Points
- When initial therapies for either menstrual pain or heavy menstrual bleeding fail, a reevaluation of the initial diagnosis is warranted.
- Care must be taken to avoid compounding side effects when adding adjunctive treatment options.
- The addition of a second therapy with a different mechanism of action is appropriate when initial treatment is insufficient.
- Hysterectomy provides the ultimate treatment for both dysmenorrhea and heavy menses, but it should remain a last resort.

References

1. De Sanctis V, Soliman A, Bernasconi S, et al. Primary dysmenorrhea in adolescents: prevalence, impact and recent knowledge. Pediatr Endocrinol Rev. 2015;13(2):512–20.
2. Derry CJ, Derry S, Moore RA. Caffeine as an analgesic adjuvant for acute pain in adults. Cochrane Database Syst Rev. 2014;(12):CD009281.
3. Lee B, Hong SH, Kim K, et al. Efficacy of the device combining high-frequency transcutaneous electrical nerve stimulation and thermotherapy for relieving primary dysmenorrhea: a randomized, single-blind, placebo-controlled trial. Eur J Obstet Gynecol Reprod Biol. 2015;194:58–63.

 4. Igwea SE, Tabansi-Ochuogu CS, Abaraogu UO. TENS and heat therapy for pain relief and quality of life improvement in individuals with primary dysmenorrhea: a systematic review. Complement Ther Clin Pract. 2016;24:86–91.
 5. Yiu KW, Chan SS, Chung TK. Mothers' attitude to the use of a combined oral contraceptive pill by their daughters for menstrual disorders or contraception. Hong Kong Med J. 2017;23(2):150–7.
 6. Harel Z, Riggs S, Vaz R, Flanagan P, Dunn K, Harel D. Adolescents' experience with the combined estrogen and progestin transdermal contraceptive method Ortho Evra. J Pediatr Adolesc Gynecol. 2005;18(2):85–90.
 7. Ling FW, For the Pelvic Pain Study Group. Randomized controlled trial of depot leuprolide in patients with chronic pelvic pain and clinically suspected endometriosis. Obstet Gynecol. 1999;93:51–8.
 8. American College of Obstetricians and Gynecologists. Management of endometriosis. Practice Bulletin No. 113. Obstet Gynecol. 2010;116:223–36.
 9. Sulak PJ, Cressman BE, Waldrop E, Holleman S, Kuehl TJ. Extending the duration of active oral contraceptive pills to manage hormone withdrawal symptoms. Obstet Gynecol. 1997;89(2):179–83.
10. Wilkinson JP, Kadir RA. Management of abnormal uterine bleeding in adolescents. J Pediatr Adolesc Gynecol. 2010;23:S22–30.
11. Lichten EM, Bombard J. Surgical treatment of primary dysmenorrhea with laparoscopic uterine nerve ablation. J Reprod Med. 1987;32:37–41.
12. Vercellini P, Aimi G, Busacca M, et al. Laparoscopic uterosacral ligament resection for dysmenorrhea associated with endometriosis: results of a randomized, controlled trial. Fertil Steril. 2003;80(2):310–9.
13. Proctor ML, Latthe PM, Farquhar CM, et al. Surgical interruption of pelvic nerve pathways for primary and secondary dysmenorrhoea. Cochrane Database Syst Rev. 2005;(4):CD001896.
14. Latthe PM, Proctor ML, Farquhar CM, Johnson N, Khan KS. Surgical interruption of pelvic nerve pathways in dysmenorrhea: a systematic review of effectiveness. Acta Obstet Gynecol Scand. 2007;86(1):4–15.
15. Webster JC. Diseases of women: a text-book for students and practitioners. Edinburgh & London: Young J. Pentland; 1898. p. 57. Fig. 29
16. Yen YK, Liu WM, Yuan CC, Ng HT. Addition of laparoscopic uterine nerve ablation to laparoscopic bipolar coagulation of uterine vessels for women with uterine myomas and dysmenorrhea. J Am Assoc Gynecol Laparosc. 2001;8(4):573–8.
17. Juang CM, Chou P, Yen MS, et al. Laparoscopic uterosacral nerve ablation with and without presacral neurectomy in the treatment of primary dysmenorrhea: a prospective efficacy analysis. J Reprod Med. 2007;52:591–6.
18. Chen FP, Chang SD, Chu KK, Soong YK. Comparison of laparoscopic presacral neurectomy and laparoscopic uterine nerve ablation for primary dysmenorrhea. J Reprod Med. 1996;41:463–6.
19. Papasakelariou C. Long-term results of laparoscopic uterosacral nerve ablation. Gynaecol Endosc. 1996;5:177–9.
20. Moawad NS, Santamaria E, Johnson M, Shuster J. Cost-effectiveness of office hysteroscopy for abnormal uterine bleeding. JSLS. 2014;18(3.) pii: e2014.00393
21. Di Spiezio SA, Spinelli M, Zizolfi B, Nappi C. Ambulatory management of heavy menstrual bleeding. Womens Health (Lond). 2016;12(1):35–43.
22. DI Spiezio Sardo A, Ceci O, Zizolfi B, Nappi C, Bettocchi S. Office myomectomy. Minerva Ginecol. 2016;68(3):321–7.
23. Wortman M. "See-and-treat" hysteroscopy in the management of endometrial polyps. Surg Technol Int. 2016;28:177–84.
24. Keyhan S, Munro MG. Office diagnostic and operative hysteroscopy using local anesthesia only: an analysis of patient reported pain and other procedural outcomes. J Minim Invasive Gynecol. 2014;21(5):791–8.

25. Cooper NA, Middleton L, Smith P, et al. OPT trial collaborative group. A patient-preference cohort study of office versus inpatient uterine polyp treatment for abnormal uterine bleeding. Gynecol Surg. 2016;13(4):313–22.
26. Duplay S, Clado S. Traité d'Hystéroscopie, Instrumentation, Technique Opératoire, Études Cliniques. Rennes: Fr. Simon, Succ De A Le Roy, Impriveur Dreveté; 1898. p. 60.
27. Davies J, Kadir RA. Heavy menstrual bleeding: an update on management. Thromb Res. 2017;151(Suppl 1):S70–7.
28. Fergusson RJ, Lethaby A, Shepperd S, Farquhar C. Endometrial resection and ablation versus hysterectomy for heavy menstrual bleeding. Cochrane Database Syst Rev. 2013;(11):CD000329.
29. Marjoribanks J, Lethaby A, Farquhar C. Surgery versus medical therapy for heavy menstrual bleeding. Cochrane Database Syst Rev. 2016;(1):CD003855.
30. Lethaby A, Vollenhoven B. Fibroids (uterine myomatosis, leiomyomas). BMJ Clin Evid. 2011;2011. pii: 0814
31. Scarperi S, Pontrelli G, Campana C, et al. Laparoscopic radiofrequency thermal ablation for uterine adenomyosis. JSLS. 2015;19(4.) pii: e2015.00071

Additional Resources

American College of Obstetricians and Gynecologists. Endometrial ablation. ACOG Practice Bulletin No. 81. Obstet Gynecol. 2007;109:1233–48.
American College of Obstetricians and Gynecologists. Alternatives to hysterectomy in the management of leiomyomas. ACOG Practice Bulletin No. 96. Obstet Gynecol. 2008;112:201–7.
Centini G, Troia L, Lazzeri L, Petraglia F, Luisi S. Modern operative hysteroscopy. Minerva Ginecol. 2016;68(2):126–32.
Davies J, Kadir RA. Heavy menstrual bleeding: an update on management. Thromb Res. 2017;151(Suppl 1):S70–7.
Gimpelson RJ. Office hysteroscopy. Clin Obstet Gynecol. 1992;35(2):270–81.
Heikinheimo O, Fraser I. The current status of hormonal therapies for heavy menstrual bleeding. Best Pract Res Clin Obstet Gynaecol. 2017;40:111–20.
Kwok A, Lam A, Ford R. Laparoscopic presacral neurectomy: a review. Obstet Gynecol Surv. 2001;56(2):99–104.
Kumar V, Chodankar R, Gupta JK. Endometrial ablation for heavy menstrual bleeding. Womens Health (Lond). 2016;12(1):45–52.
Maybin JA, Critchley HO. Medical management of heavy menstrual bleeding. Womens Health (Lond). 2016;12(1):27–34.
Ray S, Ray A. Non-surgical interventions for treating heavy menstrual bleeding (menorrhagia) in women with bleeding disorders. Cochrane Database Syst Rev. 2016;(11):CD010338.

Index

© Springer International Publishing AG 2018
R.P. Smith, *Dysmenorrhea and Menorrhagia*,
https://doi.org/10.1007/978-3-319-71964-1